Contents

Acknowledgements

The WHO Special Programme of Research, Development and Research Training in Human Reproduction wishes to acknowledge the active participation, in all stages of the compilation and editing of the third edition of the *WHO Laboratory Manual for the Examination of Human Semen and Sperm–Cervical Mucus Interaction*, of the following:

Dr R.J. Aitken
MRC Reproductive Biology Unit
Centre for Reproductive Biology
37 Chalmers Street
Edinburgh EH3 9EW
United Kingdom

Dr A. Aribarg
Department of Obstetrics and
  Gynaecology
Chulalongkorn Hospital Medical
  School
Rama 4 Road
Bangkok 10500
Thailand

Dr K. Gopalkrishnan
Institute for Research in
  Reproduction (ICMR)
Jehangir Merwanji Street
Parel
Bombay 400 012
India

Dr D.W. Hamilton
Department of Cell Biology and
  Neuroanatomy
4-135 Jackson Hall
Minneapolis, Minnesota
USA

Dr D.F. Katz
Department of Obstetrics and
  Gynecology
Division of Reproductive Biology and
  Medicine
University of California
Davis, CA 95616
USA

Dr D. Mortimer
Sydney IVF
183 Macquarie Street
Sydney, NSW 2000
Australia

Dr E. Nieschlag
Institute for Reproductive Medicine of
  the University
Steinfurterstrasse 107
D-4400 Münster
Germany

Dr C. Sekadde-Kigondu
Department of Obstetrics and
  Gynaecology
Kenyatta National Hospital
University of Nairobi
P.O. Box 19676
Nairobi
Kenya

Dr C. Wang
Divisions of Endocrinology,
  Metabolism & Reproductive
  Endocrinology
Cedars-Sinai Medical Center
444 South San Vincente Blvd
Los Angeles, CA 90048
USA

Dr C.H. Yeung
Institute for Reproductive Medicine of
  the University
Steinfurterstrasse 107
D-4400 Münster
Germany

Dr G.M.H. Waites
Special Programme of Research,
  Development and Research
  Training in Human Reproduction
World Health Organization
1211 Geneva 27
Switzerland

Valuable contributions were made to particular aspects of the present edition by the following:

Dr D.M. Phillips
Population Council
6th floor
Tower Building
1188 York Avenue at 64th Street
New York, NY
USA

Dr T.M.M. Farley, Dr P.J. Rowe, and
  Dr P.F.A. Van Look
Special Programme of Research,
  Development and Research
  Training in Human Reproduction
World Health Organization
1211 Geneva 27
Switzerland

Abbreviations

A23187	a calcium ionophore
AID	artificial insemination by donor semen
AIH	artificial insemination by husband semen
BBT	basal body temperature
BSA	bovine serum albumin (Cohn fraction V)
CASA	computer-aided sperm analysis
CFU	colony forming units
CI	colour index
DMSO	dimethyl sulfoxide
DTT	dithiotreitol
EDTA	ethylenediaminetetraacetic acid
GIFT	gamete intra-fallopian transfer
hCG	human chorionic gonadotrophin
HIV	human immunodeficiency virus
HOPT	hamster occyte penetration test
HOS	hypo-osmotic swelling test
HPF	high-power field
HSA	human serum albumin (Cohn fraction V)
HZA	hemi-zona assay
IBT	immunobead test
Ig	immunoglobulin
IU	international unit*
IVF	*in-vitro* fertilization
MAR	mixed antiglobulin reaction
NADH	nicotinamide adenine dinucleotide (reduced form)
PBS	phosphate buffered saline
PCT	post-coital test
PMS	pregnant mare's serum
PNP	para-nitrophenol
SCMC	sperm-cervical mucus contact
SMIT	sperm-mucus interaction test
SPA	sperm penetration assay (synonymous with HOPT)
TBS	tris buffered saline
TCA	trichloracetic acid
U	(international) unit*
WBC	white blood cell (leucocyte)

*IU for enzymes refers to the conversion of 1 μmole substrate per minute at 37°C.

1

Introduction

In response to a growing need for the standardization of procedures for the examination of human semen, the World Health Organization (WHO) published a *Laboratory Manual for the Examination of Human Semen and Semen–Cervical Mucus Interaction* in 1980. A second edition followed in 1987. These publications have been used extensively by clinicians and researchers worldwide. Indeed, the second edition was translated into seven languages: Arabic, Chinese, German, Indonesian, Italian, Spanish, and Russian. However, the field of andrology has continued to advance rapidly, and this, together with increased awareness of the need for standardized measurement of all semen variables, has prompted the present revision.

This third edition comes at a time of new concerns. Objective measurements in all fields of fertility regulation and in the investigation of infertility and its treatment, including assisted conception procedures, are clearly as important now as they were before. However, interest in the functional assessment of residual sperm in contraceptive efficacy studies (for example, see WHO, 1990) and the increasing concern about environmental pollutants with putative consequences for reproductive function add fresh urgency to the search for new and better standard methods of semen analysis.

For these reasons, WHO's Special Programme of Research, Development and Research Training in Human Reproduction formed a working group of experts (see Acknowledgements) to revise the manual. The present edition, with its slightly modified title *WHO Laboratory Manual for the Examination of Human Semen and Sperm–Cervical Mucus Interaction*, links with the companion *WHO Manual for the Standardized Investigation and Diagnosis of the Infertile Couple* (Cambridge University Press, in preparation).

Chapter 2 of the present manual which deals with the

1

examination of human semen is divided into three major parts. The first part describes procedures that are considered to be the minimal essential steps for semen evaluation (Section 2A: 2.1 to 2.5). The second part comprises procedures considered to be optional (Section 2B: 2.6 to 2.8), and the third part includes methods that require further evaluation and are therefore still considered to be research tools (Section 2C: 2.9 and 2.10).

Certain procedures described as optional tests in the earlier editions have been replaced by others. For example, the simplified Papanicolaou stain has been omitted and the Shorr stain has been introduced. Among the biochemical methods for the analysis of seminal plasma, the measurement of adenosine triphosphate has been deleted but the measurements of acid phosphatase and neutral α-glucosidase have been included. These changes have been made to reflect current practice in andrology laboratories. Similarly, computer-aided sperm analysis (CASA) to measure sperm motion is included in Section 2C as an example of one of a number of promising new research methods now employed in many laboratories, mostly in developed countries. While some studies suggest that CASA may be able to discriminate between semen samples of different quality, its accuracy and precision are not satisfactory and standard protocols for its use have not been finalized.

Only minor changes have been made to Chapter 3, which deals with sperm–cervical mucus interaction. On the other hand, two new chapters have been added: Chapter 4 on sperm preparation techniques and Chapter 5 on the quality control of semen analysis. These chapters are relatively brief but introduce technical and interlaboratory standardization procedures that are considered to be important and should be developed in the future.

The inclusion of new appendices – Appendix II on safety guidelines for the andrology laboratory and Appendix XXV on basic requirements for an andrology laboratory – reflects concerns for safe practice and the need for appropriate minimal equipment in the laboratory.

Finally, it should be emphasized that the major purpose of this manual is to encourage the use of standard procedures for semen analysis. This will permit improved comparability of results between laboratories and the amalgamation of data from different sources for analysis. Attention to the details of standard procedures should also sharpen the precision of results and their reproducibility. Above all, the prime objective of the earlier editions has remained: to provide a laboratory manual that will serve the needs of researchers and clinicians in developing countries.

2

Collection and examination of human semen

Normal semen is an admixture of spermatozoa suspended in secretions from the testis and epididymis which are mixed, at the time of ejaculation, with secretions from the prostate, seminal vesicles, and bulbourethral glands. The final composition is a viscous fluid that comprises the ejaculate. The collection and analysis of semen must be undertaken by properly standardized procedures if the results are to provide valid information on the fertility of the individual. This chapter and its associated appendices (III–XX) offer methods for this purpose. These methods are divided into standard, optional, and research procedures.

2A STANDARD PROCEDURES

2.1 Sample collection and delivery
The subject should be provided with clearly written or oral instructions as appropriate concerning the collection and, if required, transport of the semen sample.

(a) Ideally, the sample should be collected after a minimum of 48 hours but not longer than seven days of sexual abstinence. The name of the man, the period of abstinence, the date and time of collection, and the interval between collection and analysis should be recorded on the form accompanying each semen analysis (see Appendix X).

(b) Two samples should be collected for initial evaluation. The interval between the two collections will depend on local circumstances but should not be less than seven days or more than three months. If the results of these two assessments are markedly different, additional samples should be examined because a man's sperm output can vary considerably (Fig. 2.1).

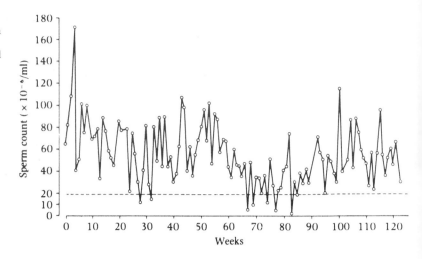

Fig. 2.1. Biweekly seminal fluid sperm concentrations from one individual over a period of 120 weeks. During this period the individual received no medication and reported no period of febrile illness. The dotted line indicates 20×10^6/ml, which is generally considered to be the lower limit of normal range (see Appendix I.A). (Unpublished data from C.A. Paulsen.)

(c) Ideally, the sample should be collected in the privacy of a room near the laboratory. If this is not possible, it should be delivered to the laboratory within one hour of collection. When the motility of the spermatozoa is abnormally low (less than 25% of spermatozoa showing rapid, progressive motility, see Section 2.4.2), the interval between collection and analysis of the second sample should be kept as short as possible. If tests of sperm function are to be performed, it is critical that the spermatozoa be separated from the seminal plasma within one hour of ejaculation (see Appendix XIX).

(d) The sample should be obtained by masturbation and ejaculated into a clean, wide-mouthed container made of glass or plastic. If plastic is used, it should be checked for possible toxic effects on spermatozoa. The container should be warm to minimize the risk of cold-shock (see (g)). If a microbiological analysis is to be done, the subject should pass urine and then wash and rinse his hands and penis before ejaculating into a sterile container (see Section 2.6).

(e) Ordinary condoms must not be used for semen collection because they can interfere with the viability of the spermatozoa. Where particular circumstances prevent collection by masturbation, special silastic condoms are available for semen collection (Zavos, 1985). Coitus interruptus is not acceptable as a means of collection because it is probable that the first portion of the ejaculate, which usually contains the highest concentration of spermatozoa, will be lost. Moreover, there will be cellular and bacteriological contamination of the sample and the acid pH of the vaginal fluid adversely affects sperm motility.

(f) Incomplete samples should not be analysed.

4

(g)   The sample should be protected from extremes of temperature (less than 20°C and more than 40°C) during transport to the laboratory.

(h)   The container should be labelled with the subject's name and with the date and time of collection.

2.2   Safe handling of specimens

Laboratory technicians should be aware that semen samples may contain harmful viruses (e.g., HIV and viruses causing hepatitis and herpes) and should therefore be handled with due care. Safety guidelines as outlined in Appendix II should be strictly observed. Good laboratory practice is fundamental to laboratory safety and cannot be replaced by special equipment (WHO, 1983).

2.3   Initial macroscopic examination

2.3.1   *Liquefaction*

A normal semen sample liquefies within 60 minutes at room temperature. In some cases, complete liquefaction does not occur within 60 minutes, and this fact should be recorded. The presence of mucous streaks, a sign of incomplete liquefaction, may interfere with the counting procedure. Normal semen samples may contain jelly-like grains (gelatinous bodies) which do not liquefy. The significance of this finding is unknown.

Occasionally, samples may not liquefy, in which case additional treatment (mechanical mixing or exposure to, e.g., bromelin 1 g/l, or plasmin 0.35–0.50 casein units/ml, or chymotrypsin 150 USP/ml) may be necessary to make the sample amenable to analysis. However, it is not known what effect this treatment may have on sperm function or on the biochemistry of seminal plasma.

The sample must be well mixed in the original container. Incomplete mixing is probably a major contributor to errors in determining sperm concentration. Continuous mixing during liquefaction by rotation of the sample container may reduce such errors (de Ziegler *et al.*, 1987).

2.3.2   *Appearance*

The semen sample should be examined immediately after liquefaction or within one hour of ejaculation, first by simple inspection at room temperature. A normal sample has an homogeneous, grey-opalescent appearance. It may appear less opaque if the sperm concentration is very low, or brown when red blood cells are present.

2.3.3 *Volume*

The volume of the ejaculate should be measured either in a graduated cylinder with a conical base or by aspirating the whole sample into a wide-mouthed pipette by means of a mechanical device (see Appendix XXV). If semen culture is to be performed or the sample is to be processed for bioassays, intrauterine insemination, or *in vitro* fertilization, sterile materials should be used in handling the samples. Plastic syringes and hypodermic needles should not be used because they affect semen analysis, particularly sperm motility.

2.3.4 *Consistency*

The consistency (often referred to as 'viscosity') of the liquefied sample can be estimated by gentle aspiration into a 5-ml pipette and then allowing the semen to drop by gravity and observing the length of the thread. A normal sample leaves the pipette as small discrete drops, while in cases of abnormal consistency the drop will form a thread more than 2 cm long. Alternatively, the consistency may be evaluated by introducing a glass rod into the sample and observing the length of the thread that forms on withdrawal of the rod. Again, the thread should not exceed 2 cm.

An abnormal consistency, e.g. because of a high mucus content, can interfere with determinations of various semen characteristics such as sperm motility and concentration, and testing for antibody coating of spermatozoa.

2.3.5 *pH*

A drop of semen is spread evenly onto the pH paper (range: pH 6.1 to 10.0). After 30 seconds, the colour of the impregnated zone should be uniform and is compared with the calibration strip to read the pH.

Whatever type of pH paper is used for this analysis, its accuracy should be checked against known standards before use.

The pH should be measured at a uniform time within one hour of ejaculation and should be in the range 7.2 to 8.0. If the pH is less than 7.0 in a sample with azoospermia, dysgenesis of the vas deferens, seminal vesicles, or epididymis may be present.

2.4 Initial microscopic investigation

During the initial microscopic investigation of the sample, estimates of the concentration, motility, and agglutination of spermatozoa and the presence of cellular elements other than spermatozoa are determined.

Although an ordinary light microscope can be used for unstained preparations, particularly if the condenser is lowered to disperse the light, a phase-contrast microscope (positive phase-contrast optics) is strongly recommended for all examinations of unstained preparations of fresh semen or washed spermatozoa.

2.4.1   *Preparation for routine semen analysis*
A fixed volume of semen (not more than 10 μl) is delivered onto a clean glass slide with a micropipette and covered with a 22 mm × 22 mm coverslip. It is important that the volume of semen and the dimensions of the coverslip are standardized so that the analyses are always carried out in a preparation of fixed depth (i.e., about 20 μm). This depth allows full expression of the rotation movement of normal spermatozoa.

The preparation is then examined at a magnification of 400 to 600 ×. The weight of the coverslip spreads the sample for optimum viewing. The freshly made wet preparation is left to stabilize for approximately one minute. Since sperm motility and velocity are highly dependent on temperature, assessment of motility should be performed as close to 37°C as possible using a warm stage or other device. The examination can be carried out at room temperature, between 20 and 24°C, and this must be standardized in the laboratory.

If the number of spermatozoa per visual field varies considerably, this indicates that the sample is not homogeneous. In such cases, the semen sample should be mixed again thoroughly. Lack of homogeneity may also result from abnormal consistency or abnormal liquefaction, from aggregation of spermatozoa in mucous threads, or from sperm agglutination. These observations should be mentioned in the semen analysis report.

If the sperm number is very low, centrifugation of the sample should be performed. A known volume of semen (as much of the ejaculate as possible) is centrifuged at 600g for 15 minutes. A known volume of the seminal plasma is then removed and the remainder is thoroughly mixed and counted as described in Section 2.5.2. The final concentration is corrected for the volume of the supernatant removed. Sperm motility and morphology assessments are also performed on the sample after centrifugation.

2.4.2   *Grading of motility*
In recent years, a number of new techniques for objectively assessing the movement characteristics of human spermatozoa have been introduced. In this manual, a simple grading system is recommended which provides the best possible assessment of sperm motility without the need for complex equipment. Laboratories interested in more detailed assessment of sperm motility are referred to Section 2.10.

The microscopic field is scanned systematically and the motility of each spermatozoon encountered is graded 'a', 'b', 'c', or 'd', according to whether it shows:

a   rapid progressive motility;

b   slow or sluggish progressive motility;

c   nonprogressive motility;

d   immotility.

The number of spermatozoa in each category can be counted with the aid of a laboratory counter. Usually four to six fields have to be scanned to classify 100 successive spermatozoa, yielding a percentage for each motility category. The count of 100 spermatozoa is repeated and the average values calculated for each category. The values are expressed as percentages, adding up to 100.

It is recommended that the motility count be repeated on a second drop of semen prepared in the same way. The results of the two counts are then averaged, provided that there is less than 10% discrepancy between them. This is simply determined by verifying that the difference between the two percentages of motile spermatozoa, i.e. the sum of classes (a), (b), and (c), is less than $\frac{1}{20}$ of their sum. For samples with less than 50% motility, the percentage of immotile spermatozoa, i.e. class (d), are used. If the difference is greater than 10%, a third preparation should be made and counted and the average percentages of the three preparations calculated and reported.

2.4.3   *Cellular elements other than spermatozoa*

The ejaculate invariably contains cells other than spermatozoa. These include polygonal epithelial cells from the urethral tract, spermatogenic cells, and leucocytes, which have been collectively referred to as 'round cells'. The concentration of such cells can be estimated in wet preparations using a suitable haemocytometer.

Leucocytes are present in most human ejaculates (Wolff & Anderson, 1988a, b; Aitken & West, 1990; Barratt *et al.*, 1990) the predominant cell type being the neutrophil. Accurate assessment of the number of leucocytes is important because the excessive presence of these cells (known as *leucocytospermia*) may indicate the existence of reproductive tract infection, which may respond to antibiotic therapy. Furthermore, leucocytospermia may be associated with defects in the semen profile including reductions in the volume of the ejaculate, sperm concentration, and sperm motility, as well as a loss of sperm function as a result of oxidative stress (Aitken *et al.*, 1989: Aitken & West, 1990) and/or the secretion of cytotoxic cytokines (Hill *et al.*, 1987).

A threshold concentration of leucocytes beyond which fertility will be impaired is difficult to define. The impact of these cells depends upon the site at which the leucocytes enter the semen, the type(s) of leucocyte involved, and their state of activation. In view of the susceptibility of human spermatozoa to oxidative stress, the presence of neutrophils is likely to be damaging, particularly if the infiltration occurs at the level of the rete testis or epididymis. Conversely, the entry of leucocytes at the moment of ejaculation, via the prostate or seminal vesicles, is probably less harmful because of the powerful antioxidant effects of seminal plasma (Jones *et al.*, 1979). As a general guide, a normal ejaculate should not contain more than 5×10^6 round cells/ml, while the number of leucocytes should not exceed 1×10^6 ml.

A number of techniques have been devised for quantifying the leucocyte population in semen. For example, biochemical criteria such as the measurement of elastase concentrations using an enzyme-linked immunosorbent assay have been found to be of value (Wolff *et al.*, 1990). In addition, Appendix III contains descriptions of two histological techniques for identifying leucocytes based on the presence of intracellular peroxidase and leucocyte-specific antigens respectively. It should be noted that the peroxidase technique gives numbers that are less than those obtained using pan-leucocyte monoclonal antibodies (Fig. 2.2).

The relationship between the number of leucocytes and the presence of genital tract infection is controversial. When the semen contains white blood cells exceeding 1×10^6/ml, microbiological tests should be performed to investigate if there is an accessory gland infection. Such tests include the examination of the first voided urine, the second voided urine, the expressed prostatic fluid, and the post-prostatic massage urine (Meares & Stamey, 1972). They also include the biochemical analysis of seminal plasma, since infection of the accessory glands often causes abnormal secretory function (Section 2.7; Comhaire *et al.*, 1980). However the absence of leucocytes does not exclude the possibility of an accessory gland infection.

The cells that are not positively identified as leucocytes include spermatids, spermatocytes, and spermatogonia. Since only spermatozoa (morphologically mature germinal cells with tails) are included in the sperm count, the concentration of other types of germinal cells or leucocytes can be calculated relative to the known number of spermatozoa.

If N is the number of a given cell type counted in the same field(s) as 100 spermatozoa and S is the sperm count in millions/ml, then

Fig 2.2. Leucocytes in human semen stained with a monoclonal antibody against the common leucocyte antigen CD45 (see Appendix III.2).

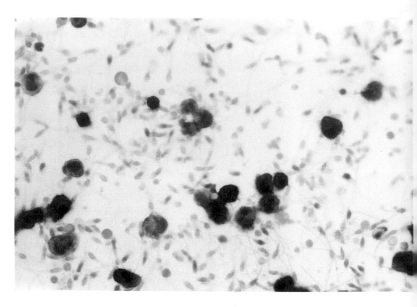

the concentration C of the given cell type in millions/ml can be calculated using the formula

$$C = \frac{N \times S}{100}$$

For example, if the number of immature germ cells counted is 10 per 100 spermatozoa and the sperm count is 120×10^6/ml, the concentration of immature germ cells is

$$\frac{10 \times 120 \times 10^6}{100} \text{ per millilitre} = 12 \text{ million per ml.}$$

2.4.4 Agglutination

Agglutination of spermatozoa means that motile spermatozoa stick to each other – head to head, midpiece to midpiece, tail to tail, or in a mixed way, e.g., midpiece to tail. The adherence either of immotile spermatozoa to each other or of motile spermatozoa to mucous threads, cells other than spermatozoa, or debris is considered to be nonspecific aggregation rather than agglutination and should be recorded as such.

The presence of agglutination is suggestive of, but not sufficient evidence for, an immunological cause of infertility. Agglutination is assessed in 10 randomly selected fields. The average percentage of spermatozoa clumped together is estimated to the nearest 5%. The extent of agglutination may be important, and even the presence of only a few groups of small numbers of agglutinated spermatozoa should be recorded. The type of agglutination should also be recorded. e.g., head to head, midpiece to midpiece, tail to tail or, when several patterns are present, mixed.

2.5 Further microscopic examinations

2.5.1 *Sperm vitality*

Sperm vitality is reflected in the proportion of spermatozoa that are 'alive' as determined by either dye exclusion or osmoregulatory capacity under hypo-osmotic conditions.

2.5.1.1 *Vital staining*

If the percentage of immotile spermatozoa exceeds 50%, the proportion of live spermatozoa should be determined by using staining techniques that are based on the principle that dead cells with damaged plasma membrane take up certain stains. Details of the protocols for performing these techniques are given in Appendix IV.

One hundred spermatozoa are counted under the light or phase-contrast microscope, differentiating the live (unstained) spermatozoa from the dead (stained) cells. These staining techniques make it possible to differentiate spermatozoa that are immotile but alive from those that are dead.

These techniques also provide a check on the accuracy of the motility evaluation, since the percentage of dead cells should not exceed the percentage of immotile spermatozoa. Furthermore, the presence of a large proportion of vital but immotile cells may be indicative of structural defects in the flagellum.

2.5.1.2 *Hypo-osmotic swelling (HOS) test*

This is a simple test based on the semipermeability of the intact cell membrane, which causes spermatozoa to 'swell' under hypo-osmotic conditions, when an influx of water results in an expansion of cell volume (Drevius & Eriksson, 1966). Introduced as a clinical test by Jeyendran *et al.* (1984), the HOS test should not be used as a sperm function test but may be used as an optional, additional vitality test. It is simple to perform and easy to score and gives additional information on the integrity and compliance of the cell membrane of the sperm tail. The method for the HOS test is given in Appendix XVIII.

2.5.2 *Counting the spermatozoa*

The concentration of spermatozoa should be determined using the haemocytometer method. In this procedure a 1:20 dilution is made from each well-mixed sample by diluting 50μl of liquefied semen with 950μl of a diluent. The latter is prepared by adding to

11

distilled water 50 g of sodium bicarbonate ($NaHCO_3$), 10 ml of 35% (v/v) formalin, and, optionally, 0.25 g of trypan blue (CI 23850) or 5 ml of saturated aqueous gentian violet, and making up the solution to a final volume of 1000 ml. The stain need not be included if phase-contrast microscopy is used.

If the preliminary examination of the semen indicates that the concentration of spermatozoa present is either excessively high or low, then the extent to which the sample is diluted should be adjusted accordingly. For samples containing less than 20×10^6 spermatozoa/ml, a 1:10 dilution may be used; for samples containing more than 100×10^6 spermatozoa/ml, a 1:50 dilution may be appropriate. White-blood-cell pipettes and automatic pipettes relying upon air displacement are *not* accurate enough for making volumetric dilutions of such viscous material as semen. A positive-displacement type of pipette should be used (see Appendix XXV).

The diluted specimen should be thoroughly mixed and a drop (10–20 μl) transferred to each chamber of an improved Neubauer haemocytometer and covered with a cover glass. The haemocytometer is allowed to stand for about 5 minutes in a humid chamber to prevent drying out. The cells sediment during this time and are then counted, preferably under a phase-contrast microscope, at a magnification of 200 to 400 ×. Only spermatozoa (morphologically mature germinal cells with tails) are counted; 'pin-heads' or tailless heads are not counted.

The procedure for counting the spermatozoa in the haemocytometer chamber is as follows. The central square of the grid in an improved Neubauer haemocytometer contains 25 large squares, each with 16 smaller squares (Fig. 2.3). For samples containing less than 10 spermatozoa per large square, the whole grid of 25 large squares should be counted; for samples containing 10 to 40 spermatozoa per large square, 10 large squares should be assessed

Fig. 2.3 The central grid of the improved Neubauer haemocytometer contains 25 squares in which the spermatozoa are to be counted (see the text and Table 2.1).

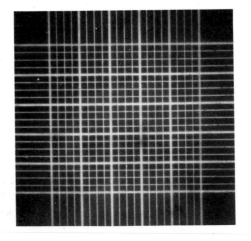

12

Table 2.1. *Correction factors for haemocytometry*

Dilution (semen + diluent)	Number of large squares counted		
	25	10	5
1 + 9	10	4	2
1 + 19	5	2	1
1 + 49	2	0.8	0.4

From Mortimer, 1985.

and, for samples containing more than 40 spermatozoa per large square, five large squares should be counted. If a spermatozoa lies on the line dividing two adjacent squares, it should be counted only if it is on the upper or the left side of the square being assessed.

Both chambers of the haemocytometer are scored and the average count calculated, provided that the difference between the two counts does not exceed $\frac{1}{20}$ of their sum (i.e., less than a 10% difference). If the two counts are not within 10%, they are discarded, the sample dilution remixed, and another haemocytometer prepared and counted.

In order to determine the concentration of spermatozoa in the original semen sample in millions/ml, divide the average number of spermatozoa by the appropriate conversion factor shown in Table 2.1. For example, if the sample has been diluted $1 + 19$, and if 162 and 170 spermatozoa have been counted in 10 large squares in each chamber, then the concentration of spermatozoa in the original semen sample is 83×10^6 ml (i.e., 166 divided by 2).

For other haemocytometers there are different correction factors that depend upon the volume of each square on the grid.

An optional procedure for determining sperm concentration employs specialized counting chambers. Although such chambers, e.g., the Makler chamber (Makler, 1980) or the Microcell (Ginsburg & Armant, 1990), are convenient in that they can be used without dilution of the specimen, they may lack the accuracy of the haemocytometer technique especially for highly viscous and/or heterogeneous specimens. If such chambers are to be used, adequate accuracy and precision must be established by comparison with haemocytometers.

2.5.3 *Analysis of the morphological characteristics of spermatozoa*
Although the morphological variability of the human spermatozoon makes differential sperm morphology counts very difficult, observations on the selection of spermatozoa recovered from the female reproductive tract (especially in postcoital cervical mucus) have helped to define the appearance of a normal spermatozoon.

Many morphologically abnormal spermatozoa have multiple defects. Previously, when multiple defects were present, only one was recorded with priority given to defects of the sperm head over those of the midpiece and to defects of the midpiece over those of the tail. However, it has been shown that the average number of defects per abnormal spermatozoon, a measure called the terato-zoospermia index, is a significant predictor of sperm function both *in vivo* and *in vitro* (Jouannet *et al.*, 1988; Mortimer *et al.*, 1990*b*). Hence, morphological assessment should be multiparametric for each spermatozoon, tallying each defect separately.

2.5.3.1   *Morphological classification of human spermatozoa*

Human spermatozoa can be classified using either bright field microscope optics on fixed, stained specimens (see Section 2.5.4 for staining methods) or high quality phase-contrast optics (total magnification at least $600 \times$) on wet preparations (Appendix V).

The heads of stained human spermatozoa are slightly smaller than the heads of living spermatozoa in the original semen, although the shapes are not appreciably different (Katz *et al.*, 1986). Strict criteria should be applied when assessing the morphological normality of the spermatozoon. The normal head should be oval in shape. Allowing for the slight shrinkage that fixation and staining induce, the length of the head should be 4.0–5.5 μm, and the width 2.5–3.5 μm. The length-to-width ratio should be 1.50 to 1.75. These values span the 95% confidence limits of comparative data for both Papanicolaou-stained and living sperm heads (Katz *et al.*, 1986). There should be a well-defined acrosomal region comprising 40–70% of the head area. There must be no neck, midpiece or tail defects, and no cytoplasmic droplet more than one-third the size of a normal sperm head. This classification scheme requires that all 'border-line' forms be considered abnormal.

Since the recommended morphological assessment considers the functional regions of the sperm cell, it is considered unnecessary routinely to distinguish between all the variations in head size and shape or between the various tail defects. However, if a region of the spermatozoon is abnormal in the majority of cells, an additional comment should be made regarding the prevalent defect(s).

The following categories of defects should be scored (see Fig. 2.4).

(a)   *Head shape/size defects*, including large, small, tapering, pyriform, amorphous, vacuolated (>20% of the head area occupied by unstained vacuolar areas), or double heads, or any combination of these.

Fig. 2.4. Spermatozoa morphology (see
2.5.3.1 and 2.5.3.2). Photomicrographs
(1000 ×) of Papanicolaou-stained
spermatozoa (see Appendix VII).
(*a*) Normal spermatozoa. N = normal.
(*b*), (*c*), (*d*), (*e*), (*f*), (*g*), (*h*), (*i*) Spermatozoa
with head, neck, midpiece, and tail defects
and pin heads. H_A = amorphous head;
H_D = double head; H_L = large head;
H_{LA} = amorphous large head;
H_P = pyriform head; H_T = tapering head;
H_V = vacuolated head; M = neck and
midpiece defect; C_D = Cytoplasmic
droplets; N = normal; P_H = pin head (these
should be counted as spermatozoa, but
noted separately); T_C = coiled tail;
T_M = multiple tail. Note that there are
white blood cells and immature germ cells
in (*d*), (*g*) (*h*) and (*i*).

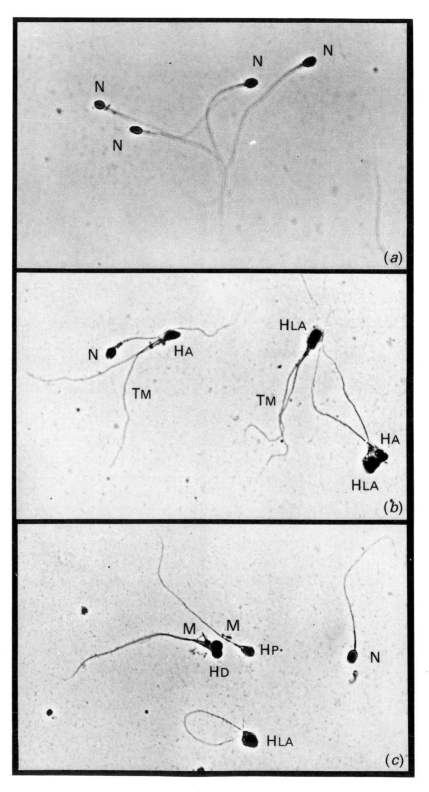

15

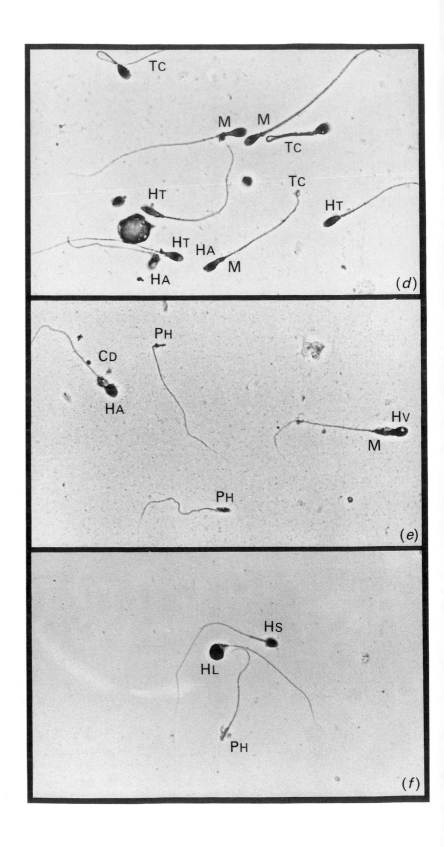

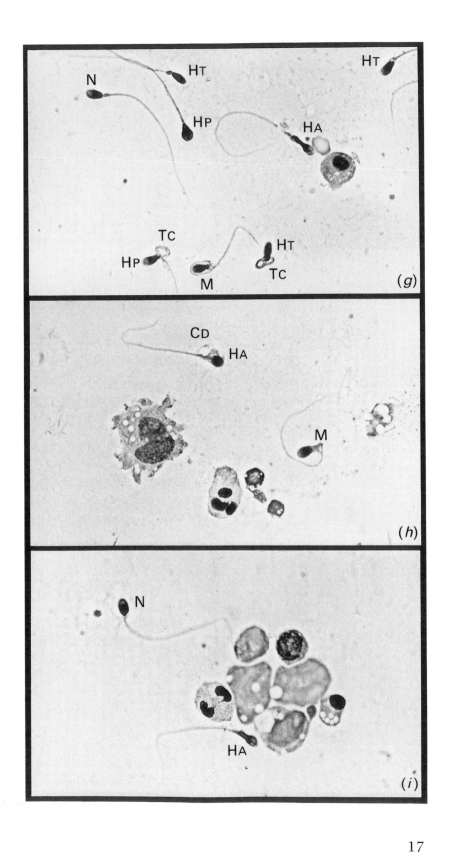

(b)   *Neck and midpiece defects*, including absent tail (seen as 'free' or 'loose' heads), non-inserted or 'bent' tail (the tail forms an angle of about 90° to the long axis of the head), distended/irregular/bent midpiece, abnormally thin midpiece (i.e., no mitochondrial sheath), or any combination of these.

(c)   *Tail defects*, including short, multiple, hairpin, broken (angulation > 90°), irregular width, or coiled tails or tails with terminal droplets, or any combination of these.

(d)   *Cytoplasmic droplets* greater than one-third the area of a normal sperm head. Cytoplasmic droplets are usually located in the neck/midpiece region of the cell, although some immature spermatozoa may have a cytoplasmic droplet at other locations along the tail.

2.5.3.2   *Performing a differential sperm morphology count*
At least 100, and preferably 200, spermatozoa are counted. With stained preparations, a $100 \times$ oil-immersion bright-field objective without a phase ring should be used.

Usually only recognizable spermatozoa are considered in a differential morphology count; immature cells up to and including the Sd_1 spermatid stage are not counted as spermatozoa. Loose or free sperm heads are counted as abnormal forms (under 'neck and midpiece defects' – see Section 2.5.3.1), but not free tails. If a high incidence of 'pinheads' is seen (> 20% incidence relative to spermatozoa), this should be noted separately; pinheads are not counted as head defects since they only rarely possess any chromatin or head structures anterior to the basal plate.

A high incidence of coiled tails may indicate that the spermatozoa have been exposed to hypo-osmotic stress, although tail coiling is also associated with sperm senescence.

2.5.3.3   *Specific 'sterilizing' defects*
In domesticated animal species, several 'sterilizing defects' have been described in which essentially all the spermatozoa produced have a specific structural defect which causes sperm dysfunction. A few similar cases have been described in men, probably the best known of which is the 'round-head defect' or 'globozoospermia'.

2.5.4   *Staining methods for human spermatozoa*
The staining can be performed using either a Giemsa method (Appendix VI), Papanicolaou stain modified for spermatozoa (Appendix VII), Bryan–Leishman stain (Appendix VIII), or Shorr stain (Appendix IX). The Giemsa stain evaluates different types of white blood cells better than spermatozoa. The Papanicolaou stain is the method most widely used in andrology laboratories. It permits staining of the acrosomal and postacrosomal regions of the head, the midpiece and tail, and can be used even for very

viscous samples. The Bryan–Leishman stain gives adequate staining of the spermatozoa; it is particularly good for the identification of immature germ cells and distinguishes them from white blood cells. The Shorr stain is simple to perform and is sufficient for evaluation of routine sperm morphology.

Although ready-to-use one-step staining procedures are available commercially, some of these stained smears cannot be stored for future reference and others do not give the same quality of smears as those suggested in this manual.

The traditional 'feathering' technique (whereby the edge of a second slide is used to drag a drop of semen along the surface of the cleaned slide) may be used to make smears of spermatozoa, but care must be taken not to make the smears too thick. Feathering works well for less viscous materials such as blood or washed sperm suspensions but is often unsuitable for viscous semen. Alternatively, one can place a drop of semen in the middle of a cleaned slide and then place a second slide, cleaned face down, on top so that the semen spreads between them; the two slides are then gently pulled apart using a sliding action to make two smears simultaneously.

The outline of all parts of the spermatozoon should be easily discernible. In Papanicolaou-stained preparations, the sperm head stains pale blue in the acrosomal region and dark blue in the postacrosomal region. The midpiece may show some red staining, but this is considered abnormal only if the midpiece is grossly distended or irregular. The tail will also be stained blue. Cytoplasmic droplets, usually located behind the head and around the midpiece, will stain green. (Fig. 2.5.)

Fig. 2.5. Papanicolaou-stained normal spermatozoa. Acrosome, pale blue; postacrosomal region, dark blue; midpiece, pale red; and tail, blue.

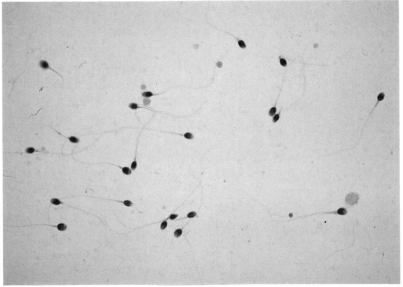

2.5.5 Testing for antibody-coating of spermatozoa

The presence of anti-sperm antibodies coating the spermatozoa is typical of, and is considered to be specific for, immunological infertility (Jones, 1986). Sperm antibodies in semen belong almost exclusively to two immunological classes: IgA and IgG. IgA antibodies might have greater clinical importance than do IgG antibodies (Kremer & Jager, 1980). IgM antibodies, because of their large molecular size, are rarely found in semen.

The screening test for antibodies is performed on the fresh semen sample and makes use of either the Immunobead method or the mixed antiglobulin reaction test (MAR test; for review see Bronson et al., 1984).

For these tests to be valid, at least 100 spermatozoa with progressive motility must be available for counting. A high mucus content of the sample may interfere with these tests. The results from the Immunobead test and the MAR test do not always agree (Scarselli et al., 1987; Hellstrom et al., 1989). The Immunobead test correlates well with sperm agglutination and immobilization tests carried out on serum. When these tests are positive, additional tests (sperm–cervical mucus contact test, sperm–cervical mucus capillary tube test, or titration of sperm antibodies in serum) will add weight and confirm the diagnosis (see Chapter 3).

2.5.5.1 Immunobead test

Antibodies present on the sperm surface can be detected by the Immunobead test (Appendix XI). Immunobeads are polyacrylamide spheres with covalently bound rabbit anti-human immunoglobulins. The presence of IgG, IgA, and IgM antibodies can be assessed simultaneously with this test.

Spermatozoa are washed free of seminal fluid by repeated centrifugation and resuspended in buffer. The sperm suspension is mixed with a suspension of Immunobeads. The preparation is examined at $400 \times$ magnification under a phase-contrast microscope. As the spermatozoa swim through the suspension, Immunobeads adhere to the motile spermatozoa that have surface-bound antibodies. The proportion of spermatozoa with surface antibodies is determined and the class (IgG, IgA, or IgM) of these antibodies can be identified by using different sets of Immunobeads (Appendix XI). Another type of Immunobead, originally intended for total B-cell labelling, can also be used as a one-step screening test for IgG, IgA, and IgM isotypes of sperm surface antibodies (Pattinson & Mortimer, 1987).

The test is considered positive when 20% or more of motile spermatozoa have Immunobead binding. However, sperm penetration into the cervical mucus and *in vivo* fertilization tend not to be significantly impaired unless 50% or more of the motile spermatozoa have antibody bound to them (Ayvaliotis *et al.*, 1985; Clarke *et al.*, 1985). On this basis, at least 50% of the motile spermatozoa must be coated with Immunobeads before the test is considered to be clinically significant. Furthermore, Immunobead binding restricted to the tail tip is not associated with impaired fertility and can be present in the semen of some fertile men.

2.5.5.2 *MAR test*
The IgG MAR test (Appendix XII) is performed by mixing fresh, untreated semen with latex particles or sheep red blood cells coated with human IgG. To this mixture is added a monospecific antihuman-IgG antiserum. The formation of mixed agglutinates between particles and motile spermatozoa proves the presence of IgG antibodies on the spermatozoa. The diagnosis of immunological infertility is probable when 50% or more of the motile spermatozoa have particles adherent. Immunological infertility is suspected when 10–50% of the motile spermatozoa have adherent particles.

2B   OPTIONAL TESTS

The tests in this part of the manual are specialized and their relevance still needs to be fully established. For this reason, they are not usually recommended for routine semen analysis.

2.6   Semen culture
Special precautions to avoid contamination need to be taken when collecting semen samples for culture. Before obtaining the sample, the subject should pass urine. Immediately afterwards, he should wash his hands and penis with soap. He should rinse away the soap and dry with a fresh, clean towel. The semen container must be sterile. For a complete examination, the sample should be given to a microbiological laboratory for tests that are not normally carried out in the andrology laboratory. The culture of seminal plasma to assess the presence of both aerobic and anaerobic organisms may help in the diagnosis of male accessory gland infection, particularly of the prostate (Mobley, 1975).

   The culture of aerobic bacteria alone can be performed with or without dilution of the semen specimen either on a dip slide or on blood agar. If the concentration of bacteria exceeds 1000 colony-forming units (CFU) per ml, the type of colonies should be examined. If the colonies appear uniform, further identification and antibiotic sensitivities should be performed by a specialized microbiology laboratory. If the colonies have different appearances, contamination should be suspected and a second semen culture should be performed with the subject carefully instructed to avoid contamination.

If the concentration of bacteria is less than 1000 CFU/ml, the culture is considered to be negative with respect to aerobic bacteria. Genital infections will require the involvement of a specialized microbiology laboratory (Brunner *et al.*, 1983; Krieger, 1984; Weidner *et al.*, 1985).

2.7 Biochemical analysis

2.7.1 *Seminal plasma*
There are various biochemical markers of accessory gland function, e.g., citric acid, zinc, γ-glutamyl transpeptidase, and acid phosphatase for the prostate gland; fructose and prostaglandins for the seminal vesicles; free L-carnitine, glycerophosphocholine, and α-glucosidase for the epididymis. A low secretory function is reflected in a low total output of the specific marker(s), which may therefore be used for the assessment of accessory gland secretory function. An infection can sometimes cause a considerable decrease in the secretory function, but despite this, the total amount of marker(s) present may still be within the wide 'normal' range. An infection can also cause irreversible damage to the secretory epithelium so that even after treatment the secretory capacity will remain low.

2.7.1.1 *Secretory capacity of the prostate*
The content of zinc and of citric acid in semen gives a reliable measure of prostate gland secretion. There are good correlations between zinc, citric acid, and prostatic acid phosphatase. The assays for these markers are given in Appendices XIII to XV.

2.7.1.2 *Secretory capacity of the seminal vesicles*
Fructose in semen reflects the secretory function of the seminal vesicles, and a method for its estimation can be found in Appendix XVI. In cases of azoospermia caused by congenital absence of the vasa deferentia, low fructose levels may indicate an associated dysgenesis of the seminal vesicles. Fructose determination is also useful in the rare cases of ejaculatory duct obstruction. The semen of men with ejaculatory duct obstruction or agenesis of the vasa

deferentia and seminal vesicles is characterized by low volume, low pH, no coagulation, and no characteristic semen odour.

2.7.1.3 *Secretory capacity of the epididymis*

Until recently L-carnitine was the most common epididymal marker used clinically, but α-glucosidase has become established lately in some clinics. There are two isoforms of α-glucosidase in the seminal plasma: the major, neutral one originates solely from the epididymis and the minor, acidic one mainly from the prostate. Neutral α-glucosidase has been shown to be more epididymal specific and sensitive than L-carnitine and glycerophosphocholine, and its measurement is therefore of better diagnostic value for distal ductal obstruction when used in conjunction with hormonal and testicular parameters. Furthermore, the assay of neutral α-glucosidase (Appendix XVII) is simpler, cheaper, and less time-consuming than those of the other two markers.

2.8 Immature germ cells

The different types of immature germ cells appearing in semen (Fig. 2.6) are usually indicative of disorders of spermatogenesis; their identification can be aided by the use of the Bryan–Leishman stain (Appendix VIII). Germ cells from semen can be used to study meiotic chromosomes and can provide material for the diagnosis of chromosomal disorders (Egozcue *et al.*, 1983).

2C RESEARCH TESTS

2.9 Sperm function tests

2.9.1 *Spermatozoa*

Understanding of the mechanisms responsible for defective sperm function has so increased that time-consuming bioassays may soon be replaced with simple biochemical tests. For example, there is now evidence that peroxidative damage, induced by the excessive generation of reactive oxygen species (for example, hydrogen peroxide), may be involved in the etiology of defective sperm function (Aitken & Clarkson, 1987; Aitken *et al.*, 1989, 1991; Alvarez *et al.*, 1987; Jones *et al.*, 1979).

Defective spermatozoa are also characterized by abnormally high activities of certain enzymes, such as creatine phosphokinase (Huszar *et al.*, 1988, 1990). The excessive generation of reactive oxygen species and the presence of high levels of creatine

Fig. 2.6.

Immature germ cells
These cells do not have tails and thus have not completed their developmental process. They are classified according to their staining and morphological characteristics. In general, their nuclei stain violet to purple and the cytoplasm is grey using Bryan–Leishman stain (see Appendix VIII).

(a)

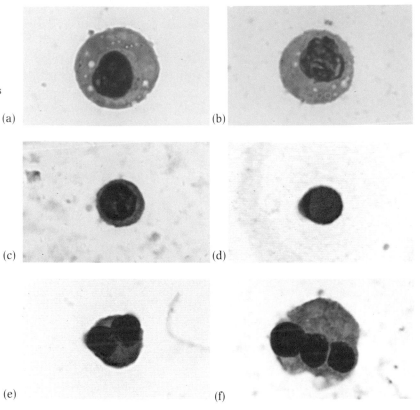

(b)

(c)

(d)

(e)

(f)

(a) *Spermatogonia*
Type A (nuclear diameter 6 to 7 μm). These cells usually contain one or two nucleoli that may be seen resting on the edge of the nucleus within characteristic 'halos'.

(b) *Primary spermatocyte*
(Nuclear diameter 8 to 9 μm.) This cell, when stained, has a large spherical, dark violet to purple nucleus in a grey cytoplasm. The nucleus is usually homogeneous, but occasionally chromatin threads are seen.

(c) *Secondary spermatocyte*
(Nuclear diameter 7 μm.) This cell stains exactly as a primary spermatocyte, but is smaller in diameter. In contrast to lymphocytes the nucleus is spherical.

(d), **(e)** and **(f)** *Spermatids*
These cells are usually spherical in shape and 4 to 5 μm in diameter. The acrosomal cap can sometimes be seen as a small magenta crescent-shaped protrusion on one side of the cell. The remainder of the cell generally stains dark purple. Several spermatids may share a common cytoplasm but are distinguished from polymorphonuclear leucocytes by the lack of granular cytoplasm, the absence of nuclear bridges and their spherical shapes. Spermatids may sometimes show the presence of fused acrosomes.

phosphokinase may both reflect a single defect in the spermatozoa characterized by abnormalities in the midpiece (Rao *et al.*, 1989).

2.9.2   *Zona-free hamster oocyte test*

A WHO consultation (1986) to examine the value of this test concluded that, when controlled and if associated with other appropriate objective measurements, e.g. of sperm motility, it might form the basis of a prediction of sperm function. The standardized protocol agreed at the consultation is given in Appendix XIX.

The ultrastructural details of sperm-oocyte fusion in the hamster oocyte penetration test are identical to those in man in that fusion with the vitelline membrane of the oocyte is initiated by the plasma membrane overlying the equatorial segment of acrosome-reacted human spermatozoa. In this respect the test is biologically meaningful. Where the test differs from the physiological situation is in the absence of the zona pellucida.

The interaction between the sperm plasma membrane and a glycoprotein constituent of the zona pellucida is responsible for triggering the acrosome reaction. In the absence of an acrosome reaction, fusion with the oocyte is impossible. The conventional hamster oocyte test depends upon the occurrence of spontaneous acrosome reactions in populations of spermatozoa incubated for prolonged periods of time *in vitro*. Since this procedure is less efficient than the biological process and may involve different mechanisms, false negative results (patients who fail in the hamster oocyte test but succeed in fertilizing human oocytes *in vitro* or *in vivo*) have frequently been recorded (WHO, 1986).

The intracellular signals that initiate the acrosome reaction following sperm–zona pellucida interaction are an influx of calcium and a cytoplasmic alkalinization. Both can be generated artificially with the divalent cation ionophore, A23187 (Aitken *et al.*, 1987, 1991; Appendix XIX).

2.9.3 *Human zona pellucida binding tests*

Recently tests have been developed to assess the binding of human spermatozoa to human zonae pellucidae. The tests make use of nonviable, nonfertilizable human oocytes from autopsy or surgically removed ovaries or from *in vitro* fertilization programmes. These oocytes can be kept in high salt solutions for several weeks (Yanagimachi *et al.*, 1979). The hemizona assay (Burkman *et al.*, 1988; Oehninger *et al.*, 1989) involves microdissection of the zona pellucida into equal halves and testing the binding on each matching half with the same number of test and control spermatozoa. Another assay differentially labels the test sample spermatozoa with one fluorescent dye (e.g., fluorescein) and the control sample with another (e.g., rhodamine, Liu *et al.*, 1988, 1989). The number of spermatozoa from the test and the control sample bound to the zona are counted and compared. Both zona binding tests have been shown to correlate with the success of *in vitro* fertilization. These tests are limited by the availability of human oocytes and the need for a minimum sperm count. The results need to be validated in a larger number of laboratories around the world.

2.9.4 *Acrosome reaction scoring*

Many techniques are available for assessing the acrosomal status of human spermatozoa. Those using fluorescent lectins, often in conjunction with the Hoechst fluorochrome H33258 as a vital stain, are probably the simplest. Peanut agglutinin labels the outer acrosomal membrane (Mortimer *et al.*, 1990*a*) while pea agglutinin labels the acrosomal matrix (Cross *et al.*, 1986). In addition to their assessment by fluorescence microscopy, lectin-labelled spermatozoa can also be counted using flow cytometry (Purvis *et al.*, 1990).

The physiological acrosome reaction (i.e., that of spermatozoa that actually fertilize oocytes) occurs on the zona pellucida after sperm binding (see Section 2.9.1). Consequently, the development of a valid bioassay remains difficult, although calcium ionophores can be used to assess the competence of populations of capacitated spermatozoa to initiate normal acrosome reactions (see Section 2.9.2).

The clinical relevance of acrosome reaction assessments and dynamics remains to be established.

2.10 Computer-aided sperm analysis (CASA)

2.10.1 *Introduction*

It is generally believed that standardized, accurate, and precise analysis of sperm motion in semen will improve the prognostic and possibly the diagnostic activity of the andrology laboratory. Video and computer vision technology has produced new instruments that are able to identify and track individual sperm cells and thence to calculate a number of parameters characterizing the 'kinematics' (i.e., the time-dependent geometry) of sperm motion (Boyers *et al.*, 1989; Katz *et al.*, 1989; Gagnon, 1990; Mortimer, 1990). Such instruments use a computer to process the electrical signal obtained by a video camera integrated to a microscope, either by direct analysis of that signal, or by analysis of the corresponding signal from a video tape recorder (Boyers *et al.*, 1989). CASA technology and usage are not yet sufficiently developed to be regarded as a routine procedure worldwide. When properly used, CASA provides improved precision of sperm motion analysis compared to subjective visual assessments, and agreement in the measurements from several laboratories can be achieved (Davis *et al.*, 1992; Davis & Katz, 1992).

2.10.2 *Sperm measures obtained by CASA*

CASA systems are designed to obtain measurements of sperm concentration, the percentage of motile sperm, and parameters characterizing the pattern and vigour of sperm-head motion along the swimming trajectory. Some systems can also be extended to measure sperm-head morphology.

The accuracy of CASA determination of sperm concentration is compromised by the cellular elements and particulate matter other than sperm that are characteristic of human semen (Boyers *et al.*, 1989). Therefore it is not currently recommended to use CASA to measure sperm concentration in human semen, although technical improvements are anticipated. For the present, the manual use of the haemocytometer is recommended (Section 2.5.2).

CASA measurement of the percentage of motile sperm is also compromised by nonsperm matter in semen, since the instrument may have difficulty in distinguishing spermatozoa from such matter. Moreover, the CASA definition of motile sperm is based solely upon achievement of a threshold of forward velocity. By contrast, visual perception of a motile spermatozoon is frequently influenced by the presence of flagellar activity, even if the cell is not swimming forward. Consequently, CASA and visual measures of percentage motility in semen are likely to be different, the former usually producing lower values (Davis & Katz, 1992). Therefore it is recommended that a direct visual estimate of percentage motility be performed (Section 2.4.2), in addition to the measure obtained in the CASA analysis.

The particular value of present CASA systems is in delineating details of sperm-head kinematics from which a number of kinematic parameters can be computed. There are standard terms for these parameters, some of which are given in Appendix XX.

3

Sperm–cervical mucus interaction

3.1 Introduction

The human uterine cervix is a thick-walled cylindrical structure, which tapers towards the cervical os. The endocervical mucosa is an intricate system of crypts that, grouped together, give an illusory impression of glands. These crypts, which consist of pockets of columnar epithelium of the cervical mucosa, may be oblique, transverse, or longitudinally directed; they never cross one another, although they may bifurcate or extend downwards. The structure of the cervical crypts varies with age, disease, and stage of the menstrual cycle.

The cervical epithelium comprises different types of secretory cells which vary in the nature and abundance of secretory granules in different parts of the cervix. Secretions from these cells contribute to the cervical mucus. The rate of mucus secretion is a function of the secretory activity and the responsiveness of the secretory cells to circulating hormones.

Ovarian hormones regulate the secretion of cervical mucus; 17β-oestradiol (oestrogens) stimulates the production of copious amounts of watery mucus, and progesterone (progestogens) inhibits the secretory activity of the epithelial cells. The amount of cervical mucus secreted shows cyclic variations. In normal women of reproductive age, the daily mucus production varies from 500 μl during mid-cycle, to less than 100 μl during other periods of the cycle. A small amount of endometrial, tubal and possibly follicular fluid may also contribute to the cervical mucus pool. In addition, leucocytes and cellular debris from the uterine and cervical epithelia are present.

Cervical mucus is, therefore, a heterogeneous secretion containing over 90% water. It exhibits a number of rheological properties – consistency, spinnbarkeit, and ferning.

Consistency is influenced by molecular arrangement and the protein and ionic concentrations of the cervical mucus. Mucus varies in consistency during the cycle from the highly 'viscous' premenstrual form (which is often cellular) to a watery consistency at mid-cycle just before ovulation. By the time ovulation is completed, the viscosity of the mucus has already begun to increase again.

Spinnbarkeit is the term used to describe the fibrosity, the threadability, or the elasticity characteristics of cervical mucus.

Ferning refers to the degree and pattern of crystallization observed when cervical mucus is dried onto a glass surface (Fig. 3.1).

Cervical mucus is a hydrogel comprising a high 'viscosity' component and a low 'viscosity' component made up of electrolytes, organic compounds, and soluble proteins. The high 'viscosity' component is a macromolecular network of mucin, which influences the rheological properties of the mucus. Cervical mucin is a fibrillar system consisting of subunits made of a peptide core and oligosaccharide side-chains. Cyclic alteration in the constituents of cervical mucus may influence sperm penetrability and survival. Sperm begin to penetrate human cervical mucus at approximately the ninth day of a normal cycle and the penetrability increases gradually to a peak just before ovulation. Sperm penetration then begins to diminish, even before large changes in mucus properties are apparent. Individual variations in time and degree of sperm penetrability are common. Motile spermatozoa may be guided by lines of strain of cervical mucus *in vivo* to the cervical crypts, where they may be retained and released at a slow rate into the uterus and fallopian tubes.

The following properties may be ascribed to the cervix and its secretion; (*a*) receptivity to sperm penetration at or near ovulation and interference with entry at other times, (*b*) protection of sperm from the hostile environment of the vagina and from being phagocytosed, (*c*) supplementation of the energy requirements of sperm, (*d*) a filtering effect (i.e., sperm selection on the basis of differential motility: see Mortimer *et al.*, 1982; Katz *et al.*, 1990), (*e*) a short-term sperm reservoir, and (*f*) the site of initiation of sperm capacitation.

Spermatozoa within the mucus are, at all times, suspended in a fluid medium. The interaction of spermatozoa with the secretions of the female reproductive tract is of critical importance for the survival and functional ability of spermatozoa. There is no practical method at present of evaluating the effects of human uterine and tubal fluids on spermatozoa, but cervical mucus is readily available for sampling and study. Evaluation of sperm–cervical mucus interaction, therefore, is an important measure to be included in any complete investigation of infertility.

3.2   Collection and preservation of cervical mucus

3.2.1   *Collection procedure*

The cervix is exposed with a speculum and the external os is gently wiped with a cotton swab to remove the external pool of vaginal contaminants. Cervical mucus is collected from the endocervical canal by any one of the following methods. The mucus can be aspirated with a tuberculin syringe (without a needle), a mucus syringe, a pipette, or a polyethylene tube. Whenever possible, the quality of the mucus should be evaluated immediately on collection. If this is not possible, the mucus should be preserved (Section 3.2.2) until it can be tested.

When mucus is collected by aspiration, it is important to standardize the manner in which suction pressure is applied to the collection device (syringe, catheter, etc.). Suction is initiated after the tip of the device has been advanced approximately 1 cm into the cervical canal. Suction is then maintained as the device is withdrawn. Just prior to withdrawal of the device from the external cervical os, suction pressure is released. It is then advisable to clamp the catheter to protect against accumulation of air bubbles or vaginal material in the collected mucus when the device is removed from the cervical canal.

When cervical mucus is inadequate in either amount or quality, its production can be increased by the administration of 20–50 μg/day ethinyloestradiol, beginning on the fifth day of a given cycle for a period of 10 days. The mucus may be collected at any time, 7–10 days after the start of administration of ethinyloestradiol. This procedure will produce a more hydrated, and therefore less viscous, mucus secretion. While this approach may be useful in assessing sperm–mucus interaction *in vitro*, it will not necessarily reflect the *in vivo* situation for the couple when hormones are not administered.

3.2.2   *Storage and preservation*

Mucus can be preserved either in the original tuberculin syringe or polyethylene tube or in small test tubes and sealed with a stopper or with paraffin paper to avoid dehydration. Care should be taken to minimize the air space in the storage container. The samples should be preserved in a refrigerator at 4°C for a period not exceeding 5 days. If possible, mucus specimens should be utilized within 2 days of collection, and the interval between collection and use should always be noted. Rheological and sperm penetration tests should not be performed on mucus specimens that have been frozen and thawed.

3.3 Evaluation of cervical mucus

Evaluation of the properties of cervical mucus includes assessment of spinnbarkeit, ferning (crystallization), consistency, and pH. Appendix XXI shows a sample form for recording the postcoital test in which these cervical mucus properties are scored according to the system devised by Moghissi (1976), based on the original proposal of Insler *et al.* (1972). The maximum score is 15. A score greater than 10 is usually indicative of a good cervical mucus favouring sperm penetration, and a score less than 10 may represent unfavourable cervical mucus. The score is derived from the volume of cervical mucus collected (Section 3.3.1) and four variables (Sections 3.3.2 to 3.3.5) describing its characteristics and appearance. The pH of the mucus is not included in the total cervical mucus score.

3.3.1 Volume

Volume is scored as follows:
0 = 0 ml,
1 = 0.1 ml,
2 = 0.2 ml,
3 = 0.3 ml or more.

3.3.2 Consistency

The consistency of cervical mucus is the most important factor influencing sperm penetration. There is little resistance to sperm migration through the cervical mucus in mid-cycle, but 'viscous' mucus such as that observed during the luteal phase forms a more formidable barrier. Cellular debris and leucocytes in cervical mucus impede sperm migration. Gross endocervicitis has been alleged to be associated with reduced fertility.

Consistency is scored as follows:
0 = thick, highly 'viscous', premenstrual mucus,
1 = mucus of intermediate 'viscosity',
2 = mildly 'viscous' mucus,
3 = watery, minimally 'viscous', mid-cycle (pre-ovulatory) mucus.

3.3.3 Ferning

Ferning (Fig. 3.1) is scored by examination of several fields around the preparation and expressed as the highest degree of ferning that is *typical* of the specimen according to the following definitions:
0 = no crystallization,
1 = atypical fern formation,
2 = primary and secondary stem ferning,
3 = tertiary and quarternary stem ferning.

Fig. 3.1. Examples of fern formation in cervical mucus air-dried on glass microscope slides (scale: × 100). Fern types can be very variable, depending on, for example, the thickness of the preparation or the number of cells present. In addition, a preparation can show more than one stage of the ferning: sometimes all stages can be found in one preparation.

(a) Score 3 ferning: a, primary stem: b. secondary stem; c. tertiary stem; d. quarternary stem
(b) Primary and secondary stems (score 2) mainly, also partially tertiary stems present.
(c) Atypical fern crystallization (score 1).
(d) No crystallization (score 0). The 'thick-walled' round structures are air bubbles.

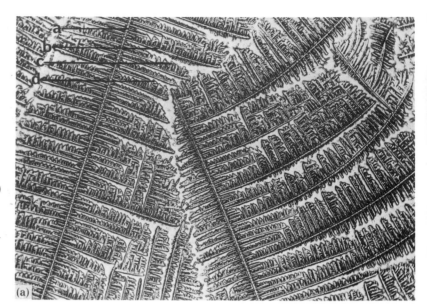

(a)

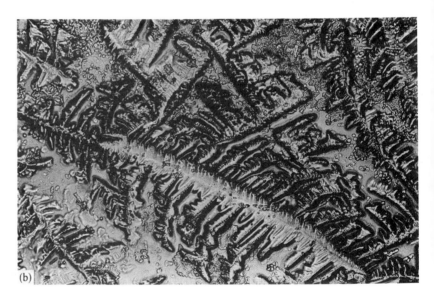

(b)

3.3.4 *Spinnbarkeit*

The cervical mucus is touched with a cover slip or a second slide held crosswise, which is lifted gently. The length of the cervical mucus thread stretched in between is estimated in centimetres and is scored as follows:
0 = < 1 cm,
1 = 1–4 cm,
2 = 5–8 cm,
3 = 9 cm or more.

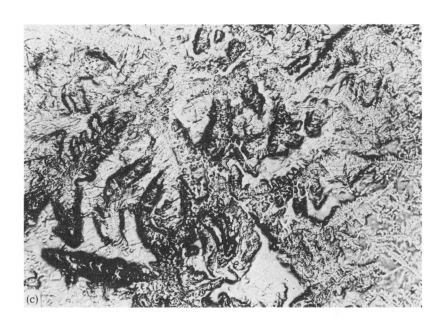

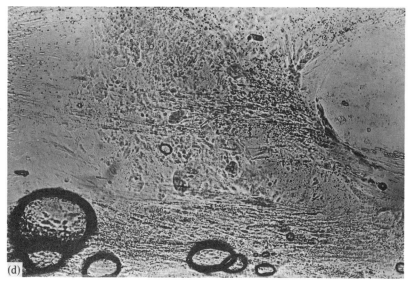

3.3.5 *Cellularity*

An estimate of the number of leucocytes and other cells in the cervical mucus is made at 400 × magnification (sometimes called high power field or HPF). Calibration of the area of a standard HPF is discussed in Appendix XXIII. The conversion factor is 10 cells/HPF equals 500 cells/mm^3 (i.e., per μl) for a standard depth of 100 μm. This is based on the use of a wide-field ocular lens with an aperture 20mm in diameter.

The rank scores for cells are:

0 = > 20 cells/HPF   or > 1000 cells/mm^3

1 = 11–20 cells/HPF   or 501–1000 cells/mm³
2 = 1–10 cells/HPF   or 1–500 cells/mm³
3 = 0 cells

3.3.6 *pH*

The pH of cervical mucus should be obtained with pH paper, range 6.4–8.0, *in situ* or immediately following collection. If the pH is measured *in situ*, care should be taken to measure it correctly, since the pH of exocervical mucus is always lower than that of mucus in the endocervical canal. Care should also be taken to avoid contamination with secretions of the vagina, which have an acidic pH.

Spermatozoa are susceptible to changes in pH of the cervical mucus. Acid mucus immobilizes spermatozoa, whereas alkaline mucus may enhance motility. Excessive alkalinity of the cervical mucus (pH greater than 8.5) may, however, adversely effect the viability of spermatozoa. The optimum pH value for sperm migration and survival in the cervical mucus is between 7.0 and 8.5, which represents the pH range of normal, mid-cycle cervical mucus. However, a pH value between 6.0 and 7.0 may still be compatible with sperm penetration.

In some cases cervical mucus may be substantially more acidic. This can be due either to abnormal secretion or to the presence of a bacterial infection (e.g., *Lactobacillus*). Such a finding must not be assumed to be an artefact.

3.4 Sperm–cervical mucus interaction

Cervical mucus is receptive to sperm migration for a limited time during the cycle. Oestrogen-influenced mucus favours penetration. The length of time during which spermatozoa can penetrate cervical mucus varies considerably from one woman to another, and may vary in the same individual from one cycle to another. This should, therefore, be evaluated for each subject to determine the optimum time for the sperm penetration tests to be performed.

3.4.1 *In vivo test (postcoital test)*
3.4.1.1 *Timing*

Postcoital tests should be performed as closely as possible to the time of ovulation as determined by clinical criteria – i.e., usual cycle length, basal body temperature, cervical mucus changes, vaginal cytology and, when available, plasma or urinary oestrogen assays and ovarian ultrasound examination. The couple should be instructed to abstain from sexual intercourse for two days prior to the day on which the test is performed. It is important for any laboratory to evaluate the mucus at a standard time after coitus. This time should be from 9 to 24 hours (Appendix XXI).

3.4.1.2   *Technique of postcoital test*
A non-lubricated speculum is inserted into the vagina and a sample of the fluid pool in the posterior vaginal fornix is aspirated with a tuberculin syringe (without needle), a pipette, or a polyethylene tube. Using a different syringe or catheter, a sample of mucus is then aspirated from the endocervical canal (Section 3.2.1), placed on a glass microscope slide, covered with a coverslip, and examined under a phase-contrast microscope. A standard depth can be achieved for this preparation by supporting the coverslip with silicone grease impregnated with glass microspheres 100 μm in diameter. This permits standardized determination of sperm concentration within the mucus (Appendix XXII).

3.4.1.3   *Vaginal pool sample*
Spermatozoa are usually killed in the vagina within two hours. The purpose of examining the vaginal pool sample is to ensure that semen has actually been deposited in the vagina.

3.4.1.4   *Cervical mucus sample*
The number of spermatozoa in the lower part of the cervical canal varies with time elapsed after intercourse. Some 2–3 hours after coitus, there is a large accumulation of spermatozoa in the lower part of the cervical canal.

It is recommended that the concentration of spermatozoa within the mucus be expressed in standard units (no. spermatozoa/mm^3), which is analogous to the measurement of mucus cellularity (Section 3.3.5). This necessitates calibrating the area of the field of view in the microscope (Appendix XXII).

Sperm motility in cervical mucus is graded as follows: (a) rapid progressive motility; (b) slow or sluggish progressive motility; (c) non-progressive motility; and (d) immotile spermatozoa (Section 2.4.2).

In a normal woman, after coitus at mid-cycle with a male partner with normal semen parameters, more than 50 motile spermatozoa (motility categories 'a' and 'b') per HPF (400 ×) are commonly observed in the endocervical specimen at 9–24 hours after coitus (Moghissi, 1976, 1986). This is equivalent to more than 2500 spermatozoa/mm^3. Twenty or more spermatozoa/HPF (> 1000/mm^3) with category 'a' directional motility may be considered satisfactory. The presence of fewer than 10 spermatozoa/HPF (< 500/mm^3), particularly when associated with the sluggish or circular motion of category 'b', is an indication of decreased sperm penetration or abnormality of the cervical mucus.

3.4.1.5   *Interpretation*
The purpose of a postcoital test is not only to determine the

number of active spermatozoa in the cervical mucus but also to evaluate sperm survival and behaviour many hours after coitus (reservoir role). Therefore, a test performed 9–24 hours postcoitally, represents the optimum time for estimating the longevity and survival of spermatozoa.

The presence of an adequate number of motile spermatozoa at this stage in the endocervix excludes cervical factors as possible causes of infertility.

The postcoital test should be repeated if the initial result is negative or abnormal. When no spermatozoa are found, the couple should be asked to confirm that ejaculation and deposition of spermatozoa into the vagina have occurred. A negative test may also be due to incorrect timing. A test performed too early or too late in the menstrual cycle may be negative in an otherwise fertile woman. In some women the test may be positive for only one or two days during the entire menstrual cycle. When ovulation cannot be timed with a reasonable degree of accuracy, it may be necessary to repeat the postcoital test several times during a cycle or to perform repeated tests *in vitro*. With these facts in mind, postcoital tests may be interpreted on a rational basis (Appendix XXI).

3.4.2 *In vitro tests*

A detailed assessment of sperm–cervical mucus interaction may be undertaken using *in vitro* penetration tests. There are three major categories of these: (1) the slide test, (2) the sperm–cervical mucus contact test, and (3) the capillary tube test. The first two techniques are simple to perform, provide useful information, and are described below as a routine component in the assessment of semen quality. The capillary tube test is a more sophisticated form of analysis that provides a semiquantitative measure of sperm penetration into the mucus. A protocol for this test is given in Appendix XXII.

In vitro tests should be done within one hour of semen collection.

When fresh, mid-cycle human cervical mucus is not available, surrogate gels may be used as an alternative for studies not directly related to infertility diagnosis. Bovine cervical mucus obtained at oestrus has some physical properties similar to mid-cycle human cervical mucus, and human spermatozoa can readily penetrate such mucus *in vitro*. However, the qualitative features of this penetration are different from those observed when human mucus is used. Bovine mucus cannot be standardized and it is not therefore a reliable alternative to human mucus.

Synthetic gels are being developed as an alternative to human cervical mucus for tests of sperm migration. Two such gels use hyaluronate (Wikland *et al.*, 1987; Mortimer *et al.*, 1990*b*) or polyacrylamide (Lorton *et al.*, 1981) as the macromolecular component. These gels do not duplicate all the features of human sperm–mucus interaction. For example, sperm penetration is not affected by the presence of antibodies on the spermatozoa, a problem also shared by bovine mucus. When such gels are drawn into a capillary tube their microstructures are not so sufficiently aligned that spermatozoa swim parallel to the long axis of the tube. Thus, qualitative standards for interpreting sperm penetration will be different from those relevant to human mucus.

3.4.2.1　*Simplified slide test*

A drop of cervical mucus is placed on a slide and flattened by a coverslip (22 mm × 22 mm). The depth of this preparation can be standardized by supporting the coverslip with silicone grease containing 100 μm glass beads (Section 3.4.1.2; Appendix XXIII). A drop of semen is deposited at each side and in contact with the edge of the coverslip so that the semen moves under the coverslip by capillary force. In this way a clear interface is obtained between the cervical mucus and semen.

The slide preparation is incubated at 37°C in a moist chamber for 30 minutes.

At the interface, finger-like projections or phalanges of seminal fluid develop within a few minutes and penetrate into the mucus. Most spermatozoa penetrate the phalangeal canal before entering the mucus. In many instances, a single spermatozoon appears to lead a column of sperm into the mucus. Once in the cervical mucus the spermatozoa fan out and move at random. Some return to the seminal plasma, while most migrate deep into the cervical mucus until they meet with resistance from cellular debris or leucocytes.

3.4.2.2　*Interpretation*

Interpretation of this test is subjective because it is impossible to standardize the size and shape of the semen–mucus interface in a plain slide preparation. Consequently, it is recommended that the test be used only as a qualitative assessment of sperm–mucus interaction.

Useful observations from the test are as follows.

(*a*)　Spermatozoa penetrate into the mucus phase and more than 90% are motile with definite progression (normal result).

(*b*)　Spermatozoa penetrate into the mucus phase but most do not progress further than 500 μm (i.e., about 10 sperm lengths) from the semen–mucus interface (poor result).

(*c*)　Spermatozoa penetrate into the mucus phase but rapidly become either immotile or show the 'shaking' pattern of movement (abnormal result).

(*d*) No penetration of spermatozoa through the semen–mucus interface takes place. Phalanges may or may not be formed, but the spermatozoa congregate along the semen side of the interface (abnormal result).

When the purpose of the test is to compare the quality of various cervical mucus specimens, a single sample of semen with optimum count, motility, and morphology should be used. On the other hand, when the interest is to evaluate the quality of several semen specimens, the same sample of cervical mucus should be used to assess the ability of spermatozoa to penetrate into it.

3.4.2.3 *The sperm–cervical mucus contact (SCMC) test*

The purpose of this test is to detect the presence of anti-spermatozoal antibodies on spermatozoa and/or in cervical mucus. The result of the test also indicates to what extent the antibodies inhibit sperm penetration and migration.

The SCMC test is performed by placing a small amount (10–50 μl) of pre-ovulatory cervical mucus and an approximately equal amount of fresh semen on one end of a microscope slide. The two materials are thoroughly mixed. Another drop of the same semen sample is placed on the other end of the slide. The semen–mucus mixture and the semen drop are covered with coverslips. The preparation is stored in a moist Petri dish at room temperature. After 30 minutes the percentage of motile spermatozoa in the semen–mucus mixture that are rapidly shaking is determined. The semen alone serves as a control for sperm activity. Immotile or slowly shaking spermatozoa are ignored. Shaking spermatozoa that are either moving slowly forward or show intermittent forward movements are considered to belong to the shaking fraction.

3.4.2.4 *Interpretation*

A high shaking percentage means that most spermatozoa cannot pass the cervical mucus and thus cannot reach the oocyte.

The results are classified as follows.
(*a*) Negative: 0–25% shaking.
(*b*) Weakly positive: 26–50% shaking (the test should be repeated).
(*c*) Positive: 51–75% shaking.
(*d*) Strongly positive: 76–100% shaking.

When a positive or strongly positive SCMC test is obtained using the husband's semen and the wife's mucus, crossover testing using donor semen and donor cervical mucus should be performed to identify whether the antibodies concerned are present in the semen or in the cervical mucus.

A high shaking percentage is in most cases due to antibodies on spermatozoa and is only occasionally due to anti-spermatozoal antibodies in cervical mucus.

When scoring an SCMC test, the percentage of immotile spermatozoa should also be recorded in order to identify other causes of sperm immobilization different from the 'shaking' phenomenon. These may include the presence of specific, complement-dependent spermotoxic antibodies either on the sperm surface or in the cervical mucus or, more commonly, a direct effect of acidic mucus upon the spermatozoa.

3.4.2.5 *The capillary tube test*
See Appendix XXII.

4

Sperm preparation techniques

A number of therapeutic and diagnostic techniques in clinical andrology depend on the separation of human spermatozoa from seminal plasma. The traditional method of sperm preparation involved a simple washing procedure during which the semen was diluted with a suitable culture medium (such as Earle's medium supplemented with 10% serum) and processed through three cycles of centrifugation ($500g$ for 5 minutes) and resuspension.

Although this technique successfully separated the spermatozoa from the seminal plasma, the repeated centrifugation (and hence compaction) of unselected cell populations, including leucocytes and defective spermatozoa, was found to disrupt the fertilizing potential of the normal spermatozoa in the same ejaculate (Aitken & Clarkson, 1988). Sperm function could, however, be maintained if the motile, functional spermatozoa were selected before the centrifugation step.

The selection of functional spermatozoa depends on their enhanced motility and higher density. Preparation procedures dependent on sperm motility include the 'swim up' procedure (Lopata *et al.*, 1976; Harris *et al.*, 1981; Makler *et al.*, 1984), in which the more motile spermatozoa are allowed to migrate out of seminal plasma into an overlying layer of culture medium, before being pelleted and washed by a single cycle of centrifugation (Aitken & Clarkson, 1988; Appendix XXIV). A variant of this is a 'swim down' procedure, in which the semen is layered on top of a column of medium, the viscosity of which has been increased by the addition of extra albumin (Urry *et al.*, 1983; Aitken & Clarkson, 1988).

Separation of functional spermatozoa by virtue of their high density (Berger *et al.*, 1985; Lessley & Garner, 1983) has been most readily achieved using simple two-step Percoll gradients (Appendix XXIV), although alternative media such as Nycodenz (Gellert-Mortimer *et al.*, 1988; Serafini *et al.*, 1990) have also been described.

5

Quality control of semen analysis

5.1 Introduction

It is in the nature of laboratory tests that they are never entirely free from errors. Understanding the source and extent of such errors is a prerequisite for correct appreciation of test results in diagnostic procedures. In order to evaluate these errors, quality control has been introduced and become routine practice in many laboratory tests. Until recently, the preconditions for quality control in the andrology laboratory were not met because of difficulties in doing analyses with live gametes as analytes and their use for standard preparations and because of the lack of definitive and reference methods for the determination of semen characteristics.

While reference methods are slowly being introduced, e.g. flow-cytometry for the estimation of sperm concentration, the world-wide use of the WHO manual over the past decade has led to a greatly increased standardization of semen analysis techniques. This has provided a basis for quality control. Several laboratories have started to introduce internal quality control as suggested by some investigators (Mortimer *et al.*, 1986; Dunphy *et al.*, 1989; Knuth *et al.*, 1989) and the first trials for external quality control are being performed (Neuwinger *et al.*, 1990). The various models for quality control require further evaluation before a general recommendation can be made, but even at this stage all laboratories should start using internal quality control schemes.

5.2 Internal quality assurance

For the purposes of internal quality assurance, aliquots of pooled semen samples can be stored and analysed at weekly intervals for sperm concentration. For sperm morphology, a number of slides can be prepared and reanalysed at intervals either by the same or different observers. To determine the precision of sperm motility estimates, different technicians may make independent observations on the same fresh sample, or aliquots of (pooled) semen samples may be cryopreserved and analysed at intervals. In the absence of semen cryobanking facilities, video recordings of semen samples may be used as surrogates.

5.3 Methodology

At the present time the precision of the techniques used should be determined by estimates of intra- and inter-technician variability at regular intervals. These measurements should consider not so much the degree of agreement between observations or between observers but rather the reasons for discrepancy between intra- or inter-individual measurements. While the coefficient of variation gives a summary of the intra- and inter-observer variability, more information can be obtained by considering (possibly graphically) the discrepancies between individual observations. Such a method is described by Bland & Altman, 1986.

Appendix IA

Normal values of semen variables

As for any laboratory test, it is preferable for each laboratory to determine its own normal ranges for each variable. For normal semen variables, specimens should be evaluated from men who have recently achieved a pregnancy, preferably within 12 months of the couple ceasing contraception.

A reasonable number (50 to 100) of such men are sometimes difficult to recruit and hence laboratories may rely on larger-scale studies published from other laboratories. However, although many of these studies contain large numbers of men, they usually do not take into account the time taken to achieve pregnancy.

To date, no significant differences have been found to indicate that racial factors may influence the lower limits of normality.

The following criteria of normality for a semen sample analysed according to the methods described in this manual are commonly used.

(See p. 44)

Standard tests

Volume	2.0 ml or more
pH	7.2–8.0
Sperm concentration	20×10^6 spermatozoa/ml or more
Total sperm count	40×10^6 spermatozoa per ejaculate or more
Motility	50% or more with forward progression (categories 'a' and 'b') or 25% or more with rapid progression (category 'a') within 60 minutes of ejaculation
Morphology	30% or more with normal forms[a]
Vitality	75% or more live, i.e., excluding dye
White blood cells	Fewer than 1×10^6/ml
Immunobead test	Fewer than 20% spermatozoa with adherent particles
MAR test	Fewer than 10% spermatozoa with adherent particles

Optional tests

α-Glucosidase (neutral)	20 mU or more per ejaculate (see Appendix XVII for the definition of U).
Zinc (total)	2.4 μmol or more per ejaculate
Citric acid (total)	52 μmol or more per ejaculate
Acid phosphatase (total)	200 U or more per ejaculate (see Appendix XV for the definition of U)
Fructose (total)	13 μmol or more per ejaculate

[a] Although no clinical studies have been completed, experience in a number of centres suggests that the percentage of normal forms should be adjusted downwards when more strict criteria are applied. An empirical reference value is suggested to be 30% or more with normal forms.

Appendix IB

Nomenclature for some semen variables

Since it is often difficult to describe all deviations for normal semen variables with words and numbers, a nomenclature was introduced to indicate the kind of alteration under discussion (Eliasson *et al.*, 1970). It is important to recognize that this nomenclature describes only some semen variables and does not imply any causal relationship. With this stipulation, the nomenclature can be used as follows:

Normozoospermia	Normal ejaculate as defined in IA
Oligozoospermia	Sperm concentration fewer than 20×10^6/ml
Asthenozoospermia	Fewer than 50% spermatozoa with forward progression (categories 'a' and 'b') or fewer than 25% spermatozoa with category 'a' movement (see Section 2.4.2)
Teratozoospermia	Fewer than 30% spermatozoa with normal morphology
Oligoasthenoterato-zoospermia	Signifies disturbance of all three variables (combinations of only two prefixes may also be used)
Azoospermia	No spermatozoa in the ejaculate
Aspermia	No ejaculate

Reference
Eliasson, R., Hellinga, F., Lübcke, F., Meyhöfer, W., Niermann, H., Steeno, O. & Schirren, C. (1970) Empfehlungen zur Nomenklatur in der Andrologie. *Andrologia.* **2**: 1257.

Appendix II

Safety guidelines for the andrology laboratory[a]

(1) All personnel working in the andrology laboratory should be vaccinated for hepatitis B, as is required for medical personnel in general.

(2) Laboratory personnel must handle every semen sample as if it were contaminated with sexually transmitted diseases or other infectious microorganisms.

(3) Strict precautions must be taken to avoid accidental wounds from sharp instruments contaminated with semen and the contact of semen with open skin lesions.

(4) Disposable rubber or plastic gloves must be worn when handling fresh and frozen semen or seminal plasma and any containers that have come into contact with semen or seminal plasma. Gloves must be removed and discarded when leaving the laboratory or handling the telephone, etc. Gloves must never be reused.

(5) A laboratory coat or disposable gown must be worn in the andrology laboratory. This coat or gown must be removed on leaving the andrology laboratory. Such clothing should never be worn in social rooms or cafeterias.

(6) Safety glasses must be worn at all times in the andrology laboratory when handling frozen semen vials (vials can explode while thawing).

(7) Hands must be washed after removing gowns and gloves. Hands must be washed thoroughly and immediately if they become contaminated with semen. All hand washing should be with a disinfectant soap and hot water.

(8) If the outside of a semen collection jar is contaminated it must be washed with a disinfectant solution (e.g., 5.25 g/l sodium hypochlorite, i.e., 5.25% diluted 1 : 10)

[a]Adapted from: Schrader, S.M. (1989) Safety guidelines for the andrology laboratory. *Fertility and Sterility*, **51**:387–9.

(9)   Disposable laboratory supplies should be used whenever possible.

(10)   All disposables should be collected in a special container and properly disposed of as for other infectious material.

(11)   All laboratory equipment that could potentially be contaminated by semen or seminal plasma must be disinfected or sterilized after a spill or after work activity is completed.

(12)   Mechanical pipetting devices must be used for the manipulation of liquids in the laboratory.

(13)   Pipetting by mouth is never permitted.

(14)   All procedures and manipulations of semen must be performed in such a way as to minimize the creation of droplets and aerosols. Surgical masks must be worn when procedures are conducted that have a high potential for creating aerosols or droplets. These procedures include centrifugation or vigorous mixing (vortexing) of open containers. Centrifuges should be covered or placed in exhaust hoods during centrifugation of biological fluids.

(15)   A well-equipped first-aid kit should always be available in the laboratory.

(16)   Laboratory work surfaces, which should be impermeable, must be decontaminated with a disinfectant (e.g., 5.25 g/l sodium hypochlorite or household bleach) immediately after any spills occur and also on completing the analyses each day.

(17)   Eating, drinking, smoking, applying cosmetics, storing food, etc. must not be permitted in the laboratory.

For further details the reader is referred to two WHO publications: *Laboratory Biosafety Manual*, Geneva, World Health Organization, 1983; and *Guidelines on the Sterilization and Disinfection Methods Effective Against Human Immunodeficiency Virus (HIV)*, 2nd ed., Geneva, World Health Organization, 1989 (AIDS Series, No. 2) p.10.

Appendix III

Methods for detecting leucocytes

The traditional method for counting leucocytes in human semen consists of using a histochemical procedure to identify the peroxidase enzyme that characterizes polymorphonuclear granulocytes (III.I). This technique has the advantage of being relatively easy to perform, but it does not detect activated polymorphs that have released their granules; nor does it detect other species of leucocyte, such as lymphocytes, that do not contain peroxidase. Such cells can be detected by immunocytochemical means (III.2).

III.1 Peroxidase stain using ortho-toluidine[a]

III.1.1 Reagents
(1) Saturated NH_4Cl, solution (250 g/l).
(2) Na_2 EDTA; 5% (50 ml/l) in phosphate buffer (pH 6.0).
(3) *Ortho*-toluidine, 0.025% (0.25 ml/l).[b]
(4) H_2O_2, 30% (300 ml/l) in distilled water.
  The working solution consists of: 1 ml of reagent (1); 1 ml of reagent (2); 9 ml of reagent (3); and one drop of reagent (4).
  This solution can be used for 24 hours after preparation.

III.1.2 Procedure
(i) Mix 0.1 ml semen with working solution to achieve a volume of 1 ml.
(ii) Shake for two minutes.
(iii) Leave for 20–30 minutes at room temperature.

[a]From Nahoum, C.R.D. & Cardozo, D (1980) Staining for volumetric count of leucocytes in semen and prostate-vesicular fluid. *Fertility and Sterility.* **34**:68–9.

[b]The International Agency for Research on Cancer (IARC) have stated that *orthotoluidine* 'should be regarded, for practical purposes, as if it presented a carcinogenic risk to humans' (*IARC Monographs on the Evaluation of the Carcinogenic Risk of Chemicals to Humans* (1982), vol. 27, suppl. 4, pp. 169–70).

(iv) Shake again.
(v) Peroxidase-positive cells stain brown, while peroxidase-negative cells are unstained.
(vi) Count in a haemocytometer chamber for leucocytes, or estimate the percentage of peroxidase positive and negative cells in a wet preparation.

III.2 Immunocytochemistry

All classes of human leucocytes express a specific antigen (CD 45) that can be detected using an appropriate monoclonal antibody (Mab; see Fig. 2.2). By changing the nature of the first antibody, this general procedure can be adapted to allow detection of the different types of leucocyte such as macrophages, neutrophils, B- or T- cells.

III.2.1 Reagents

(1) Dulbecco's phosphate buffered saline (PBS). Constituents of PBS solution:

$CaCl_2.2H_2O$	0.132 g
KCl	0.2 g
KH_2PO_4	0.2 g
$MgCl_2.6H_2O$	0.1 g
NaCl	8.0 g
Na_2HPO_4	1.15 g
Make up to 1 litre with water	

(2) Tris buffered saline (TBS: a $10 \times$ stock solution is prepared and diluted 1 : 10 immediately before use).

Constituents of $10 \times$ TBS solution:

Trizma base	60.55 g
NaCl	85.2 g
Add water, adjust to pH 8.6 with 1 M HCl (mol/l)	
Make up to 1 litre with water	

(3) Alkaline phosphatase substrate is prepared as described below and filtered.

Constituents of alkaline phosphatase substrate:

Naphthol AS-MX phosphate	2 mg
Dimethylformamide	0.2 ml
0.1 M Tris buffer (0.1 mol/l), pH 8.2[a]	9.7 ml
1 M Levamisole (1 mol/l)	0.1 ml
Fast Red TR salt, added just before use	10 mg

[a] 1.21 g of Trizma base dissolved in water, pH adjusted to 8.2 with 1 M HCl, made up to 100 ml with water.

(4) Primary antibody. A monoclonal antibody against the common leucocyte antigen, encoded CD45, and widely available commercially.

(5) Secondary antibody. Anti-mouse immunoglobulins raised in a rabbit; the dilution used will depend on antibody titre and source (e.g., 1 : 25 dilution of the Z259 antibody manufactured by DAKO).

(6) Alkaline phosphatase: anti-alkaline phosphatase complex (APAAP). Again the dilution will depend on antibody titre and source (e.g., 1 : 50 dilution of the D651 complex produced by DAKO).

III.2.2 Cell preparation
Procedure

(i) An aliquot of liquefied semen (approximately 0.5 ml) is mixed with five volumes of phosphate-buffered saline (PBS) and centrifuged at 500 g for 5 minutes at room temperature.

This procedure is repeated 2 × and the cell pellet resuspended in PBS to the original volume of the semen sample. The suspension is then diluted with two to five times its volume of PBS depending on the concentration of spermatozoa.

Two 5 μl aliquots of this cell are then air-dried onto a clean glass slide, fixed and stained immediately or wrapped in aluminium foil and stored at − 70°C for subsequent analysis.

(ii) The air-dried cells are fixed in absolute acetone for 10 minutes or in a mixture of acetone, methanol, and 400 g/l formaldehyde (in volumetric proportions 95 : 95 : 10) for 90 seconds, washed 2 × with Tris buffered saline (TBS; see III.2.1), and allowed to drain.

(iii) Each aliquot of fixed cells is covered with 10 μl of primary Mab and incubated in a humidified chamber for 30 minutes at room temperature. The slides are then washed a further $2 \times$ with TBS and allowed to drain.

(iv) The cells are covered with $10 \, \mu l$ of secondary antibody, incubated for 30 minutes in a humidified chamber at room temperature, washed $2 \times$ with TBS and drained.

(v) To each specimen is added $10 \, \mu l$ alkaline phosphatase: anti-alkaline phosphatase complex (APAAP), and the specimen is incubated for 1 hour in a humidified chamber at room temperature before being washed $2 \times$ in TBS and drained.

(vi) In order to intensify the reaction product, staining with the secondary antibody and APAAP can be repeated, with a 15-minute incubation period for each reagent.

(vii) The cells are washed $2 \times$ with TBS, drained, and incubated with $10 \, \mu l$ of alkaline phosphatase substrate for 18 minutes.

(viii) After the alkaline phosphatase colour reaction has developed, the slides are washed with TBS and finally counterstained for a few seconds with haematoxylin before being washed in tap water and mounted in Apathy's aqueous mounting medium.

Appendix IV

Sperm vitality staining techniques[a]

IV.1   Eosin alone

IV.1.1   Reagents

Eosin Y; make a 0.5% (5 g/l) solution of Eosin Y (C.I.45380) in a 0.9% (9 g/l) aqueous sodium chloride solution.

Alternatively, the standard stain can be obtained from a number of companies in different countries.

IV.1.2   Procedure

(i)   Mix one drop (10–15 μl) of fresh semen with one drop of 0.5% (5 g/l) Eosin solution on a microscope slide and cover with a coverslip.

(ii)   After one or two minutes, observe the preparation at 400 × under bright light or phase contrast.

(iii) Count unstained (live) and stained (dead) spermatozoa as described in the text.

IV.2   Eosin–Nigrosin (a modification of Blom's technique)

IV.2.1   Reagents

(1)   Eosin Y (C.I.45380, 10 g/l, i.e. 1% in distilled water).

(2)   Nigrosin (C.I.50420, 100 g/l, i.e. 10% in distilled water).

IV.2.2   Procedure

(i)   Mix one drop of semen with two drops of 1% (10 g/l) Eosin Y.

(ii)   After 30 seconds, add three drops of 10% (100 g/l) Nigrosin solution and mix.

(iii) Place a drop of the semen–Eosin–Nigrosin mixture on a clear microscope slide and make a smear. Allow to air-dry. The smears should not be too thick.

---

[a]Eliasson, R. (1977) Supravital staining of human spermatozoa. *Fertility and Sterility.* **28**:1257; Eliasson, R. (1981) Analysis of semen. In *The Testis*, ed. H. Burger & D. de Kretser. New York, Raven Press, pp. 381–99.

Appendix V

Differential sperm morphology: wet preparation

In order to perform a differential sperm morphology count on a wet preparation, it is necessary to attach the sperm to slides. A common method of doing this is to smear the sperm on a slide, allow to air dry, and then fix with ethanol (see Appendix VII.1). This procedure may lead to morphological artefacts due to osmotic damage to the cells and to extraction of components by ethanol. An approach often used to minimize artefacts is to suspend the cells in iso-osmotic solutions (or lightly fix the cells with an aldehyde fixative) and affix them to poly-1-lysine coated slides by letting them fall out of solution without drying, i.e., to form a wet preparation.

A typical protocol[a] would be as follows.

V.1   Reagents
(1)   Phosphate buffered saline (PBS)
The PBS comprises 0.8 g $NaH_2PO_4.H_2O$, 3.8 g $Na_2HPO_4.7H_2O$, and 16 g NaCl made up to 2000 ml with distilled water.
(2)   Poly-1-lysine coated slides
Poly-1-lysine coated slides are made from a solution of poly-1-lysine[b] in phosphate buffered saline by placing 10–20 μl of the solution in the centre of a small diamond-pencil-etched circle on the slide. Slides are dried, and can be kept in the refrigerator for about a week.

---

[a]Modified from: Suarez, S.S., Wolf, D.P. & Meizel S. (1986). Induction of the acrosome reaction in human spermatozoa by a fraction of follicular fluid. *Gamete Research*. 124:107–21.

[b]Poly-1-lysine can be purchased either as a lyophylized powder (specify molecular weight 70 000 to 150 000) or as a 10 mg/l solution that can be diluted to 0.1 mg/l. A more concentrated 0.5 mg/l solution of poly-1-lysine has also been used, as described in: Suarez *et al.*, 1986. The concentration that works best will depend partly on the particular batch of poly-1-lysine used and should be determined empirically.

V.2 Procedure

(i) Dilute semen to 1×10^6 cells/ml in sperm diluting fluid (see Section 2.5.2) or in phosphate buffered saline (PBS).

(ii) Place a poly-1-lysine coated slide in a moist chamber (for example a slide box with wetted hand towels). Put $\sim 10 \, \mu l$ of diluted semen in the small etched circle on the slide and cover the chamber.

(iii) Allow the sperm to settle out of solution and bind to the slide. The time needed for cells to settle out should be determined empirically the first time this procedure is used, but, with a volume as small as $10 \, \mu l$, 10 minutes should suffice.

(iv) After the sperm have settled a coverslip can be added directly. The sperm can now be viewed with phase-contrast microscopy. Under these conditions the sperm will not have been subjected to osmotic shock and the morphology should be free of preparative artefacts.

Appendix VI

Giemsa stain for spermatozoa and other cell nuclei

VI.1 Reagents
(1) Phosphate buffer, 0.066 M (mol/l.; pH 6.9).
320 ml KH_2PO_4, 9.1 g/l.
400 ml Na_2HPO_4, 11.9 g/l.
Adjust pH with NaOH and add distilled water to 1 litre.
(2) Giemsa stain solution (to be made fresh).
7 ml Romanovski-Giemsa.
160 ml phosphate buffer.

VI.2 Procedure
(i) Fix air-dried smears in methanol for at least five minutes.
(ii) Leave at room temperature for drying.
(iii) Stain in Giemsa stain solution for 30 minutes.
(iv) Rinse in phosphate buffer.
(v) Leave at room temperature for drying.

Appendix VII

Papanicolaou staining procedure modified for spermatozoa

The Papanicolaou stain distinguishes clearly between basophilic and acidophilic cell components and allows a detailed examination of the nuclear chromatin pattern. This method has therefore been used commonly for routine diagnostic cytology. However, the standard Papanicolaou method for vaginal cytology gives poor results when applied to spermatozoa. The present modified staining technique has proved useful in the analysis of sperm morphology and in the examination of immature germinal cells.

VII.1 **Preparation of specimen**
The smear should be air-dried and then fixed in equal parts of 95% ethanol (950 ml/l) and ether for 5–15 minutes.

VII.2 **Staining procedure**
Fixed smears should be stained according to the following procedure:

Ethanol 80%[a] (800 ml/l)	10 dips[b]
Ethanol 70% (700 ml/l)	10 dips
Ethanol 50% (500 ml/l)	10 dips
Distilled water	10 dips
Harris' or Mayer's haematoxylin	3 minutes exactly
Running water	3–5 minutes
Acid ethanol	2 dips
Running water	3–5 minutes
Scott's solution[c]	4 minutes
Distilled water	1 dip
Ethanol 50%	10 dips
Ethanol 70%	10 dips
Ethanol 80%	10 dips
Ethanol 90%	10 dips
Orange G6[d]	2 minutes
Ethanol 95%	10 dips

Ethanol 95%	10 dips
EA-50[d]	5 minutes
Ethanol 95%	5 dips
Ethanol 95%	5 dips
Ethanol 95%	5 dips
Ethanol 99.5% (995 ml/l)	2 minutes
Xylol-(three staining jars)	Approx. 1 minute in each

Change xylol if it turns milky. Mount at once with Depex or any mounting medium.

[a] Check the acidity of the water before preparing the different grades of ethanol. The pH should be 7.0.

[b] One dip corresponds to an immersion of about 1 second.

[c] Scott's solution (see Section VII.3.4) is used when the ordinary tap water is 'hard'.

[d] Stains and solutions: the prepared Papanicolaou stain (EA-50 and Orange G6) may be obtained commercially. The same companies usually manufacture the haematoxylin preparation.

VII.3 Preparation of stains

The commercially available stains are usually very satisfactory, but the stains may be prepared in the laboratory at a substantial saving as follows:

VII.3.1   Constituents of EA-36 equivalent to EA-50:

Eosin Y (C.I. 45380)	10g
Bismarck Brown Y (C.I.21000)	10 g
Light-Green SF, Yellowish (C.I.42095)	10 g
Distilled water	300 ml
95% Ethanol	2000 ml
Phosphotungstic acid	4 g
Saturated lithium carbonate solution (in distilled water)	0.5 ml

VII.3.1.1   Procedure
Stock solutions

(i)   Prepare separate 10% (100 ml/l) solutions of each of the stains as follows:

10 g of Eosin Y in 100 ml of distilled water.
10 g of Bismarck Brown Y in 100 ml of distilled water.
10 g of Light-Green SF in 100 ml of distilled water.

(ii)   To prepare 2000 ml of stain, mix the above stock solution as follows:

50 ml of Eosin Y
10 ml of Bismarck Brown Y
12.5 ml of Light-Green SF

(iii) Make up 2000 ml with 95% ethanol; add 4 g of phosphotungstic acid and 0.5 ml of saturated lithium carbonate solution.

(iv) Mix well and store solution at room temperature in dark-brown tightly capped bottles. The solution is stable for two to three months. Filter before using.

VII.3.2   *Constituents of Orange G6*

Orange G crystals (C.I.16230)	10 g
Distilled water	100 ml
95% ethanol	1000 ml
Phosphotungstic acid	0.15 g

VII.3.2.1   *Procedure*
Stock solution No. 1
Prepare 10% (100 ml/l) aqueous solution as follows:

(i) 10 g of Orange G crystals in 100 ml of distilled water.

(ii) Shake well and allow to stand in a dark brown bottle at room temperature for one week before using.

Stock solution No. 2 (Orange G6, 0.5% (5 ml/l) solution)
Prepare as follows:

(i) Stock solution No. 1, 50 ml.

(ii) Make up with 95% ethanol to 1000 ml.
      To prepare the final solution of 1000 ml of the stain:

(i) Add 0.15 g of phosphotungstic acid to 1000 ml of stock solution No. 2.

(ii) Mix well and store in dark-brown stoppered bottles at room temperature.

(iii) Filter before use.
      The solution is stable for two to three months.

VII.3.3   *Constituents of Harris haematoxylin without acetic acid*

Haematoxylin (dark crystals; C.I.75290)	8 g
95% ethanol	80 ml
$AlNH_4 (SO_4)_2.12H_2O$	160 g
Distilled water	1600 ml
HgO	6 g

VII.3.3.1   *Procedure for preparation of the staining mixture*

(i) Dissolve aluminium ammonium sulfate in distilled water by heating.

(ii) Dissolve haematoxylin crystals in 95% (950 ml/l) ethanol.

(iii) Add haematoxylin solution to aluminium ammonium sulfate solution.
(iv) Heat the mixture to 95 °C.
(v) Remove mixture from heat and slowly add the mercuric oxide while stirring. Solution will be dark purple in colour.
(vi) Immediately plunge the container into a cold water bath and filter when the solution is cold.
(vii) Store in dark-brown bottles at room temperature and allow to stand for 48 hours.
(viii) Dilute the required amount with an equal part of distilled water and filter again.

VII.3.4   *Constituents of Scott's solution*

$NaHCO_3$	3.5 g
$MgSO_4.7H_2O$	20.0 g
Distilled water	1000 ml

Scott's solution is to be used only when the ordinary tap water is 'hard' and should be changed frequently, e.g., after rinsing 20 to 25 slides.

VII.3.5   *Constituents of acid ethanol solution*

Ethanol 99.5%	300 ml
Concentrated HCl	2.0 ml
Distilled water	100 ml

Appendix VIII

Bryan–Leishman stain for sperm morphology smears

Note: Use freshly made air-dried smears from fresh samples on clean slides.

10% Alcohol formalin (100 ml/l)	1 minute	Fresh each time
80% Ethanol (800 ml/l)	5 minutes	Change every third time[a]
70% Ethanol (700 ml/l)	5 minutes	Change every third time
50% Ethanol (500 ml/l)	5 minutes	Change every third time
Alpha-naphthol	4 minutes	Change every three days

(Add 0.4 ml of 3% (30 ml/l) hydrogen peroxide to 200 ml of alpha-naphthol just prior to initial use; the solution is active for three days at room temperature.)

Running tap water	5 minutes	Running slowly
Pyronin Y	4 minutes	Fresh each week
Running tap water	3 dips[b]	Running slowly
Sodium citrate buffer	3 minutes	pH 7.5; fresh each time
Distilled water	1 minute	Fresh each time
Modified Bryan's stain	15 minutes	Fresh every other time
1% (10 ml/l) acetic acid (glacial)	2 dips	Running slowly
Running tap water	1 minute	Running slowly
Buffer and Leishman's stain	30 minutes	Fresh each time

(Filter 80 ml of Leishman's stock solution, add 100 ml buffer (pH 6.8), filter again immediately before use.)

Running tap water	1–2 dips	Running slowly
Air dry (do not blot)		

[a] Change after every 30 slides if you are using a staining jar that holds 10 slides.
[b] Each dip should be of approximately 1 second duration.

VIII.1 Special considerations

(1) Pyronin Y, modified Bryan's and Leishman's stains should be filtered prior to initial use. In addition, the buffer and Leishman's working stain should be filtered prior to use to remove precipitating stain.

(2) The final stain intensity can be increased by staining for a longer time in the buffered Leishman's stain or can be decreased by repeated washing. Check for the desired intensity with a microscope before mounting the slide.

(3) Hydrogen peroxide deteriorates rapidly in the presence of light; thus, the stock 3% solution should be stored in an amber bottle and in the dark.

(4) The stock Leishman's stain should be aged before use by storing for seven days at room temperature in the dark followed by incubation at 25–37 °C for two days in the dark. The aged solution is stable for a month if kept in a sealed container in the dark.

VIII.2 Preparation of solutions:

VIII.2.1 Bryan's stain (modified)

(i) Combine the following:
1500 ml of 1% glacial acetic acid,
0.5 g of Eosin yellow (C.I.45380),
0.5 g of Fast Green FCF (C.I.42053),
0.5 g of Naphthol Yellow S (C.I. 10316).

(ii) Mix thoroughly and store in a tightly stoppered bottle.

(iii) Filter before use.

VIII.2.2 Leishman's blood stain: stock solution

(i) Combine 0.5 g of eosinated methylene blue (a mixture of eosin Y and methylene blue, C.I.52015) and 300 ml of absolute methyl alcohol.

(ii) Mix thoroughly and allow to age in the dark at room temperature for seven days.

(iii) At the end of this time, place the stain in an incubator (35–37 °C) for two days.

(iv) After this period the stock solution is ready for use and should be stored in a tightly stoppered dark bottle, away from heat and light. Alternative blood stain stock solutions are Jenner's blood stain or Wright's blood stain, which can be obtained from any commercial house supplying standard chemicals. The timing involved with these stains must be varied at the 'Leishman's' step in the procedure, however, to achieve comparable results.

Buffer

Combine two pH 6.8 buffer tablets with 200 ml of distilled water. If not used at once, recheck pH before use.

VIII.2.3 Leishman's blood stain: working solution

(i) Just before use, combine 80 ml of filtered stock solution with 100 ml of buffer at pH 6.8.

(ii)   Alcoholic formalin: combine 10 ml of 37% formaldehyde solution with 90 ml of 95% ethanol; 0.1 g of calcium acetate may be added per 200 ml of solution to ensure a neutral pH of 7.0

(iii)   Alpha-naphthol: dissolve 1 g of alpha-naphthol in 100 ml of 40% ethanol. Immediately before initial use, add 0.2 ml of 3% hydrogen peroxide solution.

(iv)   Pyronin Y: combine 0.1 g of pyronin (C.I.45005), 4 ml of aniline, and 96 ml of 40% ethanol.

(v)   Sodium citrate buffer: mix 7 g of sodium citrate with 1 litre of 0.9% NaCl and adjust pH to 7.5.

Appendix IX

Shorr stain for sperm morphology smears

IX.1 Preparation of smear

(1) Smear about 20 μl of the sample (at $50-100 \times 10^6$ spermatozoa/ml) on a clean slide and allow to dry.

(2) Fix the smear in 75% ethanol (750 ml/l) for about 1 minute.

IX.2 Staining procedure

running water	12–15 dips
haematoxylin	1–2 minutes
running water	12–15 dips
ammonium alcohol	5 passages of 5 minutes each
running water	12–15 dips
50% ethanol (500ml/l)	5 minutes
Shorr stain	3–5 minutes
50% ethanol	5 minutes
75% ethanol (750 ml/l)	5 minutes
95% ethanol (950 ml/l)	5 minutes
absolute ethanol	2 passages of 5 minutes each
xylol	2 passages of 5 minutes each

IX.3 Reagents

(1) Haematoxylin Papanicolaou No. 1 (Merck, Darmstadt, Germany, Reference 9253).

(2) Ammonium alcohol
95 ml 75% ethanol + 5 ml 25% (250 ml/l) ammonium hydroxide

(3) Either Shorr solution (Merck, Reference 9275)

or BDH Shorr powder	4g
50% ethanol	220 ml
glacial acetic acid	2.0 ml

Dissolve powder in warm alcohol and allow it to cool.
Add the acetic acid in a fume hood and filter.

Appendix X

Sample record form for semen analysis

This sample record form is offered as a model to be adapted to different circumstances. It contains a suggested layout for recording the observations made during the semen analysis using the methods described in this manual. When used for clinical purposes, it may be useful to add certain derived variables, which are combinations of results from the data. An example of such a variable is the total motile sperm count (obtained by multiplying the sperm concentration, the semen volume, and the percentage motile sperm). Such derived variables have not been included on the sample form since their use depends on the clinical circumstances and the clinician's views of their relevance. When used for research purposes, data from the sample record form can be entered directly into a computer database, and any derived variables can be most easily (and accurately) computed electronically.

The sample record form has been printed with multiple columns for recording the results of semen analyses collected on different dates. This is a convenient way of presenting serial semen sample results, but it may not be practicable for the laboratory technicians who complete the forms. Similarly additional space may be required in certain places to allow the recording of comments and observations that cannot be coded on the form.

SAMPLE RECORD FORM FOR SEMEN ANALYSIS

	Day	Month	Year	Day	Month	Year	Day	Month	Year
Date of sample	⎣_⎮_⎮_⎮_⎮_⎮_⎦			⎣_⎮_⎮_⎮_⎮_⎮_⎦			⎣_⎮_⎮_⎮_⎮_⎮_⎦		
Duration of abstinence (days)	⎣_⎮_⎦			⎣_⎮_⎦			⎣_⎮_⎦		
Interval between ejaculation and start of analysis (min)	⎣_⎮_⎮_⎦			⎣_⎮_⎮_⎦			⎣_⎮_⎮_⎦		
Appearance (1 – normal, 2 – abnormal)	⎣_⎦			⎣_⎦			⎣_⎦		
Liquefaction (1 – normal, 2 – abnormal)	⎣_⎦			⎣_⎦			⎣_⎦		
Consistency (1 – normal, 2 – abnormal)	⎣_⎦			⎣_⎦			⎣_⎦		
Volume (ml)	⎣_⎮_⎮.⎮_⎦			⎣_⎮_⎮.⎮_⎦			⎣_⎮_⎮.⎮_⎦		
pH	⎣_⎮.⎮_⎦			⎣_⎮.⎮_⎦			⎣_⎮.⎮_⎦		
Motility (100 spermatozoa)									
(a) rapid progression	⎣_⎮_⎮_⎦			⎣_⎮_⎮_⎦			⎣_⎮_⎮_⎦		
(b) slow progression	⎣_⎮_⎮_⎦			⎣_⎮_⎮_⎦			⎣_⎮_⎮_⎦		
(c) non-progressive motility	⎣_⎮_⎮_⎦			⎣_⎮_⎮_⎦			⎣_⎮_⎮_⎦		
(d) immotile	⎣_⎮_⎮_⎦			⎣_⎮_⎮_⎦			⎣_⎮_⎮_⎦		
Agglutination (%)	⎣_⎮_⎮_⎦			⎣_⎮_⎮_⎦			⎣_⎮_⎮_⎦		
Vitality (% live)	⎣_⎮_⎮_⎦			⎣_⎮_⎮_⎦			⎣_⎮_⎮_⎦		
Concentration (10^6/ml)	⎣_⎮_⎮_⎮.⎮_⎦			⎣_⎮_⎮_⎮.⎮_⎦			⎣_⎮_⎮_⎮.⎮_⎦		
Morphology (%)									
– normal	⎣_⎮_⎮_⎦			⎣_⎮_⎮_⎦			⎣_⎮_⎮_⎦		
– head defects	⎣_⎮_⎮_⎦			⎣_⎮_⎮_⎦			⎣_⎮_⎮_⎦		
– neck or midpiece defects	⎣_⎮_⎮_⎦			⎣_⎮_⎮_⎦			⎣_⎮_⎮_⎦		
– tail defects	⎣_⎮_⎮_⎦			⎣_⎮_⎮_⎦			⎣_⎮_⎮_⎦		
– cytoplasmic droplets	⎣_⎮_⎮_⎦			⎣_⎮_⎮_⎦			⎣_⎮_⎮_⎦		
White blood cells (10^6/ml)	⎣_⎮_⎮.⎮_⎦			⎣_⎮_⎮.⎮_⎦			⎣_⎮_⎮.⎮_⎦		
Immature germ cells (10^6/ml)	⎣_⎮_⎮.⎮_⎦			⎣_⎮_⎮.⎮_⎦			⎣_⎮_⎮.⎮_⎦		
Immunobead test (% with adherent Ig beads)	⎣_⎮_⎮_⎦			⎣_⎮_⎮_⎦			⎣_⎮_⎮_⎦		
MAR test (% with adherent particles)	⎣_⎮_⎮_⎦			⎣_⎮_⎮_⎦			⎣_⎮_⎮_⎦		
Biochemistry									
zinc (mmol/l)	⎣_⎮.⎮_⎮_⎦			⎣_⎮.⎮_⎮_⎦			⎣_⎮.⎮_⎮_⎦		
citric acid (mmol/l)	⎣_⎮_⎮.⎮_⎦			⎣_⎮_⎮.⎮_⎦			⎣_⎮_⎮.⎮_⎦		
acid phosphatase (kU/l)	⎣_⎮_⎮_⎦			⎣_⎮_⎮_⎦			⎣_⎮_⎮_⎦		
fructose (mmol/l)	⎣_⎮_⎮.⎮_⎦			⎣_⎮_⎮.⎮_⎦			⎣_⎮_⎮.⎮_⎦		
α-glucosidase (neutral) (U/l)	⎣_⎮_⎮.⎮_⎦			⎣_⎮_⎮.⎮_⎦			⎣_⎮_⎮.⎮_⎦		

65

Appendix XI

Immunobead test[a]

XI.1 Reagents

(1) Immunobeads: anti-IgG, IgA and IgM beads are obtainable from BioRad Laboratories (BioRad Chemical Division, 15111 San Pablo Avenue, Richmond, CA 94806, USA) (Catalogue Nos. 170-5100, -5114, and -5120 respectively). For screening purposes, anti-Ig combined beads (170-5106), which will identify all the isotypes, can be used. Reconstitute the Immunobeads in 10 ml of Buffer I (see below) and store at $+4\,°C$. These can be kept for about one month.

(2) Stock buffer: Tyrode's solution or Dulbecco's phosphate buffered saline (PBS) can be used.

Tyrode's solution		Dulbecco's PBS	
	(g/l)		(g/l)
$CaCl_2$	0.2	$CaCl_2$	0.1
KCl	0.2	KCl	0.2
NaH_2PO_4	0.05	KH_2PO_4	0.2
$MgCl_2.6H_2O$	0.2	$MgCl_2.6H_2O$	0.1
NaCl	8.0	NaCl	8.0
$NaHCO_3$	1.0	$Na_2HPO_4.7H_2O$	2.16
Glucose	1.0		

The solution should be passed through a millipore (22μm filter) before use.

[a]Bronson, R.A., Cooper, G.W. & Rosenfeld, D. (1982) Detection of sperm specific antibodies on the spermatozoa surface by immunobead binding. *Archives of Andrology.* 9:61; Bronson, R.A., Cooper, G.W. & Rosenfeld, D. (1984) Sperm antibodies: their use in infertility. *Fertility and Sterility.* 42:171–83; Clarke, G.N. (1990) Detection of antisperm antibodies using Immunobeads. In *Handbook of the Laboratory Diagnosis and Treatment of Infertility*, ed. B.A. Keel & B.W. Webster, pp. 177–92, CRC, Boca Raton, Florida.

(3)   Buffer I: contains 0.4% (4 g/l) bovine serum albumin (BSA: Cohn fraction V): weigh out 0.4 g BSA and make up to 100 ml with stock buffer.

(4)   Buffer II: contains 5% (50 g/l) BSA: weigh out 5.0 g BSA and make up to 100 ml with stock buffer.

(5)   All solutions should be passed through a 0.22 μm or 0.45 μm millipore filter before use.

XI.2   Procedure

(i)   For each Immunobead type, add 0.2 ml of stock bead suspension to 10 ml of Buffer I in separate conical base centrifuge tubes.

(ii)   Transfer the required amount of semen to a conical base centrifuge tube and make up to 10 ml with Buffer I. The amount of semen required is determined from the sperm concentration and motility according to the following table:

Concentration (10^6/ml)	Motility (categories (a) + (b),),%^{a}	Semen required (ml)
> 50		0.2
20–50	> 40	0.4
20–50	< 40	0.8
< 20	> 40	1.0
< 20	< 40	2.0

^{a} See Section 2.4.2.

(iii)   Centrifuge the tubes at about 500 g for 5–10 minutes.

(iv)   Sperm tube(s): decant and discard the supernatant. Gently resuspend the sperm pellet in 10 ml of fresh Buffer I and centrifuge again at about 500 g for 5–10 minutes.

(v)   Immunobead tube(s): decant and discard the supernatant. Gently resuspend the beads in 0.2 ml of Buffer II.

(vi)   Sperm tube(s): decant and discard the supernatant. Gently resuspend the sperm pellet to its original aliquot volume using Buffer II.

(vii)   Place 5 μl drops of each type of Immunobead on one or more glass slides. Add 5 μl of the washed sperm suspension to each of the bead drops and mix well using either a pipettor tip or the edge of a coverslip. Place a coverslip (20 to 24 mm square) on each of the mixtures and after leaving the slide for 10 minutes in a moist chamber, observe at 400 $\times$ to 500 $\times$ magnification under a phase-contrast microscope.

(viii) Score separately the percentage of *motile* spermatozoa that are attached to Immunobeads in preparation. Count at least 100 motile spermatozoa per preparation. Record the class (IgG or IgA) and the site of binding of the Immunobeads to the spermatozoa (head, midpiece, tail, or tail-tip).

The test is regarded as positive if 20% or more of motile spermatozoa are attached to the beads and clinically significant if 50% or more of motile spermatozoa are coated with beads. Binding restricted to the tail-tip is not considered to be clinically significant.

XI.3   **Indirect Immunobead test**
This modification is used to detect anti-sperm antibodies in serum, seminal plasma, or bromelin-solubilized cervical mucus.

(i)   Normal donor spermatozoa are washed twice with Buffer I as described in XI.2 steps (ii), (iii), (iv), and (vi) above.

(ii)   The washed sperm suspension is then adjusted to a concentration of 50×10^6/ml in Buffer II.

(iii) Dilute 10 μl of the test fluid with 40 μl of Buffer II and then mix with 50 μl of the washed sperm suspension. Incubate at 37 °C for one hour.

(iv)   The spermatozoa are then washed twice again as in XI.2 steps (iii), (iv), and (vi) and the tests performed as described in steps (vii) and (viii).

XI.4   **Controls**
A positive control and a negative control should be included in each test run. A positive control can be prepared using serum from a donor (e.g., vasectomized men) with high titres of serum sperm antibodies as detected by the indirect Immunobead test. This serum is prepared as in XI.3 and assayed in parallel with each test run.

Appendix XII

Mixed antiglobulin test (MAR test)

Since IgA antibodies almost never occur without IgG antibodies, testing for the latter is sufficient as a routine screening method. In the MAR test (Ortho SpermaMAR kit from Fertility Technologies Inc. Natick, MA, USA), this is done as follows.

10 μl of unwashed fresh semen, 10 μl of IgG-coated latex particles (from Fertility Technologies Inc.) or of IgG-coated sheep blood cells, and 10 μl of antiserum to human IgG (from Hoechst-Behring ORCM-04/05, or Dakopatts A089, Denmark) are placed on a microscope slide.

The drops of semen and IgG-coated particles are mixed first, and then the drop of antiserum is admixed using a larger coverslip (e.g., 40 mm × 24 mm), which is then laid on the mixture. The wet preparation is observed under the microscope at 400 × or 600 × magnification either under bright light or phase contrast after 2–3 minutes and again after 10 minutes.

In the absence of coating antibodies, the spermatozoa will be seen swimming freely between the particles, which themselves adhere to each other in groups, proving the effectiveness of the preparation.

If sperm antibodies are present on the spermatozoa, the motile spermatozoa will have latex particles adhering to them. The motile spermatozoa are initially seen moving around with a few or even a bunch of particles attached. Eventually, the agglutinates become so massive that the spermatozoa can only move on the spot if they are attached to the particles.

At least 100 motile spermatozoa should be counted. The percentage of the motile spermatozoa that have particles attached is calculated.

Appendix XIII

Measurement of zinc in seminal plasma

XIII.1   **Background**

This colorimetric assay was developed for the determination of zinc in serum, plasma, cerebrospinal fluid, and urine. Recently, zinc values in human seminal plasma obtained by this assay were found to correlate well with those obtained by flame atomic absorption spectroscopy, suggesting that this colorimetric assay can be useful for the determination of zinc in seminal plasma in laboratories lacking atomic absorption facilities.[a]

XIII.2   **Stability of the reagents**

The kit of reagents is stable for several years at temperatures below 25 °C (obtainable from: Wako Pure Chemical Industries Ltd.)

XIII.3   **Preparation and stability of the chromogen solution**

Mix colour reagents A and B in the ratio 4:1 (e.g., 20 ml of colour reagent A and 5 ml of colour reagent B). This chromogen solution is stable for one week at 2–10 °C, and for two days at room temperature.

XIII.4   **Sample preparation**

The semen sample is centrifuged for 20 minutes at 2000 g. The seminal plasma is decanted and diluted 1:200 (e.g. 10 μl of seminal plasma added to 1.99 ml of distilled water). It should be stored in a freezer until analysis.

Note – A trichloroacetic acid (TCA) precipitation step for proteins is unnecessary because of the high dilution of seminal plasma before the colour reagent is added.

[a]Johnsen, Ø. & Eliasson, R. (1987) Evaluation of a commercially available kit for the colorimetric determination of zinc in human seminal plasma. *International Journal of Andrology*, 10:435–40.

XIII.5 Zinc standard

Zinc standard is provided by the manufacturer as a 30.6 μmol/l solution.

XIII.6 Assay procedure

Wavelength	560 nm
Cuvettes	1 cm light path
Incubation temperature	20–25 °C

(1) Put into separate test tubes 0.5 ml of water (blank), 0.5 ml of zinc standard, and 0.5 ml of diluted seminal plasma.

(2) Add 2.5 ml of working chromogen solution to each tube.

(3) Mix well, allow the mixtures to stand at room temperature for 5 minutes, and measure the absorbance within an hour at 560 nm, using the blank value as reference.

The relation between absorbance (A) and zinc concentration in seminal plasma is linear up to at least 7 mM (mmol/l).

XIII.7 Calculation

Zinc concentration in seminal plasma is calculated according to the formula:

$$\text{Concentration of zinc (mmol/1)} = \frac{A\ \text{sample}}{A\ \text{standard}} \times \frac{30.6 \times 200}{1000}$$

where 30.6 is the concentration of the zinc standard in μmol/l and 200 is the dilution factor of seminal plasma.

XIII.8 Normal values

2.4 μmol or more per ejaculate.

Appendix XIV

Determination of citric acid in seminal plasma

XIV.1 Reagents

XIV.1.1   *Boehringer Kit No. 139076 (ultraviolet method)*
One kit is sufficient for 30 determinations.
The kit contains:
   (1)   *Bottle 1* (mainly NADH): Reconstitute solution 1 by adding 12 ml of distilled water; store at $-20\,°C$ (stable for four weeks).
   (2)   *Bottle 2* (citrate-lyase): Reconstitute solution 2 by adding 0.3 ml of distilled water; store at $-20\,°C$ (stable for four weeks).

XIV.1.2   *TRA buffer (pH 7.7)*
   (i)   Dissolve 14.9 g of tri-ethanolamine in 750 ml of distilled water. Adjust to pH 7.6 by adding concentrated HCl.
   (ii)   Dissolve 0.027 g of $ZnCl_2$ in 250 ml of distilled water. Be sure that the $ZnCl_2$ is completely dissolved.
   (iii)   Add the $ZnCl_2$ solution to the tri-ethanolamine solution.
   (iv)   Add 0.5 g of sodium azide.

XIV.2 Procedure

XIV.2.1   *Preparation of seminal plasma*
Centrifuge the ejaculate at $3000\,g$ for 15 minutes or $2000\,g$ for 20 minutes.

XIV.2.2   *Extraction*
   (i)   Add 0.1 ml of seminal plasma to 4.95 ml of 15% (150 ml/l) trichloroacetic acid (TCA).
   (ii)   Add 0.75 ml 6M NaOH.
        The pH must exceed 7. If necessary add NaOH to make alkaline. The extract must be clear,

XIV.2.3   *Measurement*

   (i)   Add in a measuring cuvette:
      0.5 ml of solution 1,
      2.3 ml of TRA buffer,
      0.2 ml of seminal plasma extract.

   (ii)   Mix and measure absorption at 340 nm. Absorbance A_1.

   (iii)   Add 20 μl of solution 2.

   (iv)   Mix, and wait exactly 5 minutes.

   (v)   Measure absorption. Absorbance value A_2.

XIV.3   Calculation

Concentration of citric acid in mM (mmol/l)

$$= \frac{(A_1 - A_2)}{\text{Extinction coefficient}} \times \text{Extraction dilution}$$
$$\times \text{Absorbance dilution}$$

$$= \frac{(A_1 - A_2)}{6.3} \times 58 \times \frac{3.02 \text{ ml}}{0.2 \text{ ml}}$$
$$= (A_1 - A_2) \times 139$$

XIV.4   Normal values

52 μmol or more per ejaculate.

Appendix XV

Measurement of acid phosphatase in seminal plasma[a]

XV.1 Reagents

(1) Citrate buffer, 0.09 M (mol/l) with pH 4.8.

   Dissolve 1.73 g anhydrous free citric acid in distilled water, adjust the pH to 4.8 with 1 M NaOH and make up to 100 ml with water. Store at 4 °C.

(2) 0.1 M NaOH.

(3) *p*-Nitrophenol phosphate (substrate) solution.

   Prepare freshly each day. Calculate the volume of substrate needed and dissolve the required amount of *p*-nitrophenol phosphate disodium salt in citrate buffer to a concentration of 4 mg/ml (100μl substrate per measurement, e.g., 8 mg in 2 ml for duplicate measurements of 8 samples and a blank) or use Sigma 5 mg tablets when accurate weighing of small amounts of substrates is not possible.

(4) *p*-Nitrophenol (PNP), 5 mM (mmol/l), stock solution for standard curve. Dissolve 0.0695 g PNP in distilled water, warm the solution if necessary, and make up to 100 ml in a volumetric flask. Store at 4 °C.

(5) Sodium bisulfate ($NaHSO_4.H_2O$, 12 g/l water).

XV.2 Method

(i) Not more than 30 minutes after liquefaction, centrifuge the ejaculate at 3000 *g* for 10 minutes to separate the spermatozoa. If the sample is not assayed immediately, pipette 20 μl seminal plasma into 20 μl sodium bisulfate solution in an Eppendorf tube (pH of mixture should be betweeen 5 and 6) to stabilize the acid phosphatase during storage at room temperature for a few hours, at 4 °C for a few days, or at -20 °C for several months.

[a]Modified from Heite, H.-J. & Wetterauer, W. (1979) Acid phosphatase in seminal fluid: method of estimation and diagnostic significance. *Andrologia*. 11:113–22.

(ii) Dilute seminal plasma 10 000 times for the assay, i.e., for a stabilized sample (already diluted 1:1), dilute 10 μl into 0.5 ml citrate buffer and further dilute 10 μl of this into 1 ml buffer.

(iii) To control the assay, take two pools of stabilized seminal plasma, stored at $-20\,°C$, one containing high and the other low acid phosphatase activities previously assayed, dilute them and assay them in parallel with the samples.

(iv) Put 0.1 ml substrate solution in each assay tube and warm for 5 minutes at $37\,°C$. Add 10 μl of diluted sample and incubate at $37\,°C$ for exactly 30 minutes. Tubes without sample are also incubated as blanks.

(v) Stop the enzyme reaction by adding 1 ml NaOH solution and read the absorbance at 405 nm against the assay blanks.

(The use of tartrate to differentiate other acid phosphatases from the prostatic enzyme is generally not necessary because of the extremely high activity of the latter.)

Prepare and read PNP standard curve just before reading the samples.

Put 400 μl 5 mM (mmol/l) stock solution into a 20-ml volumetric flask and make up to 20 ml with 0.1 M (mol/l) NaOH (this solution is 100 μM i.e., μmol/l).

Dilute this 100 μM solution with 0.1 M NaOH to give standards of 0, 20, 40, 60, 80, and 100 μM and read the absorbances.

XV.3 Calculation

1 unit acid phosphatase $= 1$ μmol PNP produced per minute at $37\,°C$.

Slope of standard curve (S) = absorbance unit per μM

Net absorbance of sample (A) = absorbance measured $-$ absorbance of blank

Factor (F) = total incubation volume $\div$ sample volume $\div$ 30 minutes $\times$ dilution factor of seminal plasma
$$= 1110 \div 10 \div 30 \times 10000$$

Acid phosphatase activity in seminal plasma

$$= (A \div S) \times F \text{ mU/ml}$$
$$= (A \div S) \times F \div 1000 \text{ U/ml}$$
$$= (A \div S) \times 37 \text{ U/ml}$$

Total activity = U/ml $\times$ volume of ejaculate in ml
$$= \text{U per ejaculate}$$

Normal value: 200 U per ejaculate or more.

Appendix XVI

Determination of fructose in human seminal plasma[a]

XVI.1   Reagents
  (1)   1.8% (18g/l) $ZnSO_4.7H_2O$.
  (2)   0.1 M NaOH.
  (3)   *Indol-reagent*: 200 mg of benzoic acid is added to 100 ml of distilled water and dissolved by repeated shaking in a hot water bath (about 60 °C). When all benzoic acid is dissolved, 25 mg of indol is added. The solution is filtered and stored at 4 °C.
  (4)   *Stock fructose standard* (2.8 mM): 50.4 mg of fructose is dissolved in 100 ml of distilled water. Can be stored frozen in suitable samples.
  (5)   *Working fructose standard*: on the day of analysis, one portion of the stock standard is diluted to 0.28 mM and 0.14 mM, respectively.

XVI.2   Seminal plasma preparation
  (i)   Dilute seminal plasma 1:50 by adding 0.1 ml of seminal plasma to 4.9 ml of distilled water.
  (ii)   Add 1 ml of the diluted seminal plasma to a centrifuge tube.
  (iii) Add 0.3 ml of 18 g/l zinc sulphate: mix.
  (iv)   Add 0.2 ml of NaOH and mix thoroughly.
         (Total dilution of seminal plasma is $50 \times (1 + 0.3 + 0.2)$ ml ÷ 1 ml, i.e. 75 times)
  (v)   Let the tube stand for 15 minutes and centrifuge at 2000 g for 20 minutes.
  (vi)   Use 0.5 ml of the clear supernatant for analysis.

XVI.3   Experimental procedure
  (i)   Take four glass tubes with glass stoppers. Into the first put 0.5 ml of the supernatant from the diluted and deproteinised seminal plasma, into the second 0.5 ml of 0.28 mM working fructose

[a]Karvonen, M.J. & Malm, M. (1955) Colorimetric determination of fructose with indol. *Scandinavian Journal of Clinical Laboratory Investigation*, 7:305–307.

standard, into the third 0.5 ml of 0.14 mM fructose standard, and into the fourth 0.5 ml of distilled water (reagent blank).

(ii) Add to each tube 0.5 ml of indol reagent and 5.0 ml of concentrated HCl.[b]

(iii) Stopper the glass tubes and incubate for 20 minutes at 50 °C.

(iv) Cool in ice water to room temperature and read the absorbance at 470 nm.

XVI.4 Calculation

Fructose concentration (mmol/l) in seminal plasma $= A_s \times F \times \phi$ where A_s is the absorbance of the sample of seminal plasma, ϕ is the dilution (volume fraction) of the sample, and F is the mean fructose standard factor, according to the formula:

$$F = \tfrac{1}{2}\left(\frac{0.14}{S_1} + \frac{0.28}{S_2}\right)$$

where S_1 and S_2 are the mean absorbance readings for the 0.14 mM and 0.28 mM fructose standards, respectively. The dilution factor ϕ of the seminal plasma is 75 (see XVI.2).

XVI.5 Normal values

13 μmol or more per ejaculate.

[b]If the use of concentrated HCl is considered unpleasant, an alternative but more expensive enzymatic assay using ultraviolet spectrophotometry (e.g., Boehringer-Mannheim kit No. 139106) may be performed.

Appendix XVII

Determination of neutral α-glucosidase in seminal plasma

In most previous clinical studies, total enzyme activity at pH 6.8 was measured. In addition to the neutral isoenzyme originating from the epididymis, seminal plasma also contains an acid isoenzyme which is contributed by the prostate and can be selectively inhibited (Paquin *et al.*, 1984). The following assay improves the specificity of α-glucosidase measurement as an epididymal marker (Cooper *et al.*, 1990).

XVII.1 **Reagents**

(1) Phosphate buffer pH 6.8 (0.1 M) containing 1% sodium dodecyl-sulfate (SDS) inhibitor of acidic α-glucosidase.

   Mix 12 ml K_2HPO_4 (0.2 M) and 13 ml KH_2PO_4 (0.2 M), and make up to about 40 ml with distilled water. Adjust pH to 6.8 by adding more KH_2PO_4 when pH is more than 6.8 or more K_2HPO_4 when pH is less than 6.8. Make up final volume to 50 ml and store at 4 °C. Just before use, dissolve SDS in the volume of buffer needed (e.g., 50 mg for 5 ml).

(2) *p*-Nitrophenol glucopyranoside (PNPG; substrate, 5 g/l buffer); the required volume is freshly made for each assay.

   Add the right amount of PNPG to the required volume of reagent 1 (e.g., 25 mg/5 ml). Warm and stir on a hot plate at 50 °C for about 10 minutes to dissolve.

(3) Castanospermine (1 mM; α-glucosidase inhibitor).

   10 mM stock: dissolve 1 mg castanospermine in 0.53 ml distilled water and store at −20 °C.

   1 mM solution: add 0.1 ml 10 mM stock to 0.9 ml distilled water and store 0.2 ml aliquots at 4 °C. Spare aliquots can be stored at −20 °C.

(4) Na_2CO_3 (0.1 M)

   Dissolve 6.20 g $Na_2CO_3.H_2O$ in 500 ml distilled water.

(5) *p*-Nitrophenol (PNP; 5 mM; for standard curve); make up a fresh solution every 3 months.

Dissolve 0.0695 g PNP in distilled water, warm the solution if necessary and make up to 100 ml in a volumetric flask. Store at 4 °C in brown bottle.

XVII.2 Method
(i) Prepare water bath at 37 °C for incubation.
(ii) Thaw out and vortex sperm-free seminal plasma stored at − 20 °C.
(iii) Prepare PNPG solution (2×100 μl for each sample or blank).
(iv) Put duplicate 10 μl seminal plasma (using positive displacement pipette) into 100 μl PNPG in Eppendorf tubes and vortex.
(v) As water blank: 10 μl water into 100 μl PNPG.
(vi) As internal standards for interassay control: 10 μl from a pool of seminal plasma with high glucosidase content and 10 μl from a pool with low glucosidase content and put each into 100 μl PNPG.
(vii) As semen blanks: put 10 μl seminal plasma from pools of high and low glucosidase content (or the same individual sample) each into 100 μl PNPG. Add 5 μl castanospermine to each.
(viii) Vortex each tube and incubate for 4 hours in water bath at 37 °C (accurate temperature and incubation time are crucial).
(ix) Stop incubation by adding 1 ml 0.1 M Na_2CO_3 to each tube and vortex.
(x) Transfer 250 μl from each tube to a 96-well plate and read the absorbence at 405 nm, using the water blank to set zero.
(xi) Prepare PNP standard curve (less than 1 hour before reading absorbence). Put 400 μl 5 mM stock solution into a 20 ml volumetric flask and make up to 20 ml with 0.1 M Na_2CO_3 (this solution is 100 μM). Dilute this 100 μM (μmol/l) solution with 0.1 M Na_2CO_3 to give standards of 0, 20, 40, 60, 80, and 100 μM and read the absorbances.

XVII.3 Calculation
1 unit α-glucosidase = 1 μmol PNP produced per minute at 37 °C.
Slope of standard curve (S) = absorbance unit/μM
Net absorbance of sample (A) = absorbance − mean semen blanks
Factor (F) = total volume ÷ sample volume ÷ 240 minutes = 0.46

Neutral α-glucosidase activity in sample $= \dfrac{A}{S} \times F$ mU/ml

Total activity = mU/ml × volume of ejaculate = mU/ejaculate

XVII.4 Normal values:
20 mU per ejaculate or more
Note – The volumes used in the above method (total volume 1.1 ml) are for users of 96-well plate reader and Eppendorf tubes.

These volumes can be proportionally adjusted when different spectrophotometer cuvettes and incubation tubes are used, and the appropriate corrections must be made for the calculation of results.

References

Cooper, T.G., Yeung, C.H., Nashan, D., Jockenhövel, F. & Nieschlag, E. (1990) Improvement in the assessment of human epididymal function by the use of inhibitors in the assay of α-glucosidase in seminal plasma. *International Journal of Andrology*. **13**:297–305.

Paquin, R., Chapdelaine, P., Dube, J.Y. & Tremblay, R.R (1984) Similar biochemical properties of human seminal plasma and epididymal α-1,4-glucosidase. *Journal of Andrology*. **5**:277–82.

Appendix XVIII

Hypo-osmotic swelling test for sperm[a]

XVIII.1 **Swelling solution**

Dissolve 0.735 g sodium citrate $Na_3C_6H_5O_7.2H_2O$ and 1.351 g fructose in 100 ml distilled water. Store aliquots of this solution frozen at $-20\,°C$. Thaw and mix well before use.

XVIII.2 **Method**

Warm 1 ml swelling solution in a closed Eppendorf tube at 37 °C for about 5 minutes. Add 0.1 ml liquefied semen and mix gently with the pipette. Keep in 37 °C for at least 30 minutes (but not longer than 120 minutes) and examine the sperm cells with phase-contrast microscope. Swelling of sperm is identified as changes in the shape of the tail, as shown in Fig. XVIII.1. Repeat twice the score of swollen sperm in a total of 100 sperm counted and calculate the mean score.

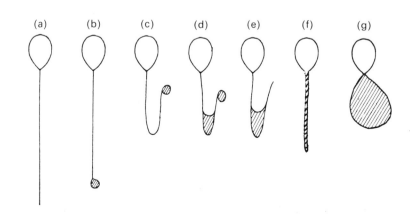

Fig. XVIII.1. Schematic representation [a] of typical morphological changes of human spermatozoa subjected to hypo-osmotic stress: a = no change; b–g = various types of tail changes. Tail region showing swelling is indicated by the hatched area.

(a) (b) (c) (d) (e) (f) (g)

[a]Jeyendran, R.S., Van der Ven, H.H., Perez-Pelaez, M., Crabo, B.G. & Zaneveld, L.J.D. (1984) Development of an assay to assess the functional integrity of the human sperm membrane and its relationship to other semen characteristics. *Journal of Reproduction and Fertility.* 70:219–28.

Appendix XIX

Protocols for the zona-free hamster oocyte test

XIX.1 **Standard protocol**

XIX.1.1 *Procedure*

(i) Allow 30 to 60 minutes for full liquefaction of the semen to occur.

(ii) The culture medium for the test is medium BWW (Biggers *et al.*, 1971). This medium is prepared as a stock solution (see Table) that can be stored at 4 °C for several weeks without deterioration. On the day of the test, a 100-ml sample of the medium stock solution is supplemented with 210 mg of sodium bicarbonate, 100 mg of glucose, 0.37 ml of a 600 g/l sodium lactate syrup, 3 mg of sodium pyruvate, 350 mg of Fraction V bovine serum albumin, 10 000 units penicillin, 10 mg streptomycin sulfate and 20 mmol/l HEPES salts. The medium should be warmed to 37 °C before use, preferably in an atmosphere of 5% CO_2, 95% air.

Components of the medium BWW stock solution used in the zona-free hamster oocyte test

Compound	Quantity
NaCl	5.540 g/l
KCl	0.356 g/l
$CaCl_2.2H_2O$	0.250 g/l
KH_2PO_4	0.162 g/l
$MgSO_4.7H_2O$	0.294 g/l
Phenol red	1.0 ml/l

(iii) Semen samples are prepared for this test using the sperm preparation techniques described in Appendix XXIV. If the 'swim-up' procedure is used, a number of tubes (three to ten depending on the volume of the sample and the concentration of the spermatozoa in semen) can be prepared.

The tubes are incubated at 37 °C for one hour in an atmosphere of 5% CO_2, 95% air. If such an incubator is not available, the tubes

(iv) may be tightly capped and maintained at 37 °C in air. During the incubation period the most motile spermatozoa migrate from the seminal plasma into the overlying medium (see page 99).

(iv) Following centrifugation at 500 g for 5 minutes, the sperm pellet is resuspended at approximately 10×10^6 spermatozoa/ml in a volume of not less than 0.5 ml and incubated for 18–24 hours at 37°C in an atmosphere of 5% CO_2, 95% air. If a CO_2 incubator is not available, the tubes can be capped tightly and incubated at 37°C in air. During the incubation period, the tubes should be inclined at an angle of 20° to the horizontal in order to prevent settlement of the spermatozoa into a pellet and

(v) to increase the surface area for gaseous exchange.

random or from mature hamsters injected on day one of the estrous cycle. Pregnant mare's serum (PMS) and human chorionic gonadotrophin (hCG) are injected intraperitoneally at a dose of 30 to 40 IU, 48 to 72 hours apart. The oocytes should then be recovered within 18 hours after the injection of hCG and prepared at room temperature using 0.1% (1 g/l) hyaluronidase and 0.1% (1 g/l) trypsin to remove the cumulus cells and zonae pellucidae respectively. Each enzyme treatment should be followed by two washes in medium BWW. The isolated oocytes can be warmed to 37 °C and introduced immediately into the sperm suspensions or stored at 4 °C for up to 24 hours.

(vi) At the end of the capacitation phase, the incubation tubes are returned to a vertical position for 20 minutes to allow settlement of any immotile cells, after which the motile spermatozoa are aspirated in the supernatant and adjusted to a fixed concentration of 3.5×10^6 motile spermatozoa/ml. The spermatozoa are then placed under liquid paraffin in 50 to 100 μl droplets, and 30 zona-free hamster oocytes are introduced, incorporating at least 15 oocytes per droplet. The gametes are then incubated at 37 °C in an atmosphere of 5% CO_2, 95% air for three hours.

(vii) The number of spermatozoa that have entered the oocytes is then assessed by carefully removing the oocytes and washing them free of loosely adherent spermatozoa; after which they are compressed to a depth of about 30 μm beneath a 22 mm × 22 mm coverslip and examined by phase-contrast microscopy. (Fixation and storage of the oocytes in, for example, 1% (10 ml/l) glutaraldehyde, followed by staining with lacmoid or aceto-orcein, is also a possibility.)

(viii) The oocytes should then be examined to determine the percentage that have spermatozoa within their cytoplasm and the mean number of incorporated spermatozoa per oocyte (Fig. XIX.1). The presence of spermatozoa remaining bound to the surface of the oocyte after the initial washing procedure should also be recorded,

Fig. XIX.1. A zona-free hamster oocyte containing human spermatozoa, as seen by phase-contrast microscopy. The arrows indicate the presence of decondensing sperm heads within the ooplasm (scale: × 500). From Aitken *et al.* (1983).

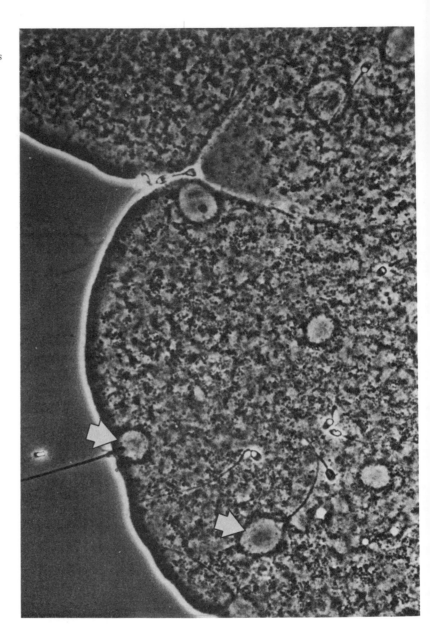

since this may give some indication of the proportion of the sperm population that has undergone the acrosome reaction.

XIX.2 Protocol incorporating Ca ionophore (A23187)

A highly motile sperm population is prepared by Percoll gradient centrifugation employing a two-step discontinuous gradient as described in Appendix XXIV. The pellet at the base of the 80%

fraction is then taken up into 8 ml of medium BWW, centrifuged at 500 g for 5 minutes and finally resuspended at a concentration of 5×10^6 motile spermatozoa/ml.

A23187 is prepared as follows: a 1 mM (mmol/l) suspension of the free acid of A23187 is prepared from a 10 mM stock in dimethylsulfoxide (DMSO) by a 1 in 10 dilution with medium BWW. This suspension is kept at 4 °C for *at least 3 days* before use.

On the day of the test, the A23187 is added to the spermatozoa to achieve two final concentrations of 1.25 and 2.5 μM (μmol/l). The dose-response curve for ionophore treatment varies from individual to individual, and as a result it is preferable to test each patient at both 1.25 and 2.5 μM. The spermatozoa are incubated with the ionophore for 3 hours, after which the cells are pelleted by centrifugation at 500 g and resuspended in the same volume of fresh medium BWW.

At this point the percentage of motile spermatozoa is assessed, and the concentration of spermatozoa is readjusted to 3.5×10^6 motile spermatozoa/ml before being dispersed as 50–100 μl droplets under paraffin oil. However, valid results can still be obtained using concentrations as low as 1×10^6 motile spermatozoa/ml (Aitken & Elton, 1986)

Zona-free hamster oocytes are prepared as described by Yanagimachi *et al.* (1976) and dispensed into the droplets, at an incidence of about 5 oocytes/drop and 20 oocytes/sample.

After a further 3 hours the oocytes are recovered from the droplets, washed free of loosely adherent spermatozoa, compressed to a depth of about 30 μm under a 22×22 mm coverslip on a glass slide and assessed for the presence of decondensing sperm heads with an attached or closely associated tail, using phase-contrast microscopy. The number of sperm penetrating each egg is assessed and the results expressed as the mean number of spermatozoa penetrating each oocyte.

XIX.3 Quality control

The assays must be performed with an adequate degree of quality control. The within-assay coefficient of variation should be established by replicating the analysis of a single sample at least 10 times in one assay. Under such circumstances the within-assay coefficient of variation should not exceed 15%. The between-assay coefficient of variation should not exceed 25% and can be ascertained using a cryostored pool of spermatozoa with a known level of penetration. Any assay in which the value obtained for the standard preparation is more than two units of standard deviation away from the mean value should be rejected as unreliable. Any analysis in which a penetration score of zero is obtained should be repeated on a separate semen sample.

References

Aitken, R.J. & Elton, R.A. (1986) Application of a Poisson-gamma model to study the influence of gamete concentration on sperm-oocyte fusion in the zona-free hamster egg penetration test. *Journal of Reproduction and Fertility.* **78**: 733–39.

Aitken, R.J., Templeton, A., Schats, R., Best, F., Richardson, D., Djahanbakhch, O. & Lees, M. (1983) Methods of assessing the functional capacity of human spermatozoa: their role in the selection of patients for *in vitro* fertilization. In *Fertilization of the Human Egg* in vitro, ed. H. Beier & H. Lindner. Berlin, Springer, pp. 147–65.

Biggers, J.D., Whitten, W.K. & Whittingham, D.G. (1971) The culture of mouse embryos *in vitro*. In *Methods in Mammalian Embryology*, ed. J.C. Daniel, San Francisco, Freeman, pp. 86–116.

Yanagimachi, R., Yanagimachi, H. & Rogers, B.J. (1976) The use of zona-free animal ova as a test system for the assessment of fertilizing capacity of human spermatozoa. *Biology of Reproduction.* **15**:471–6.

Appendix XX

Computer-aided sperm analysis (CASA)

XX.1 Preparation of the semen for application in a CASA instrument

In general, the criteria for semen collection and handling for CASA applications are identical to those specified in Section 2A for visual analysis. The CASA system must include provision for the maintenance of specimen temperature at 37 °C because the parameters of sperm motion are temperature sensitive.

Current CASA systems have difficulty in continuously identifying individual spermatozoa when the concentration is greater than approximately 40×10^6 spermatozoa/ml (Vantman *et al.*, 1988). Thus, such specimens require dilution if accurate measurements are to be achieved. The preferred diluent is fresh, homologous seminal plasma, which can be obtained by gentle centrifugation. Sometimes it is not possible to obtain fresh, homologous seminal plasma. For example, highly viscous semen specimens preclude the simple extraction of a liquid seminal plasma component. Heterologous, pooled and/or cryostored seminal plasma cannot be standardized, and may have deleterious effects upon fresh semen. Therefore it is recommended that isotonic artificial medium, pH 7.2–7.5, be used for semen dilution, if fresh homologous plasma is not available. Dulbecco's phosphate-buffered saline solution is suitable for this purpose. If the initial sperm concentration is $\geq 100 \times 10^6$ spermatozoa/ml, then supplementation of the medium with bovine serum albumin (0.3 g/l) and glucose (1 g/l) may prevent alterations in sperm motion due to dilution.

A standard microscope slide preparation must be used. For the analysis of semen, application of $7\,\mu l$ of material to a slide, which is covered with a $22\ mm \times 22\ mm$ coverglass is acceptable. This achieves a depth of approximately $15\ \mu m$ in the preparation. Special chambers which provide a fixed specimen depth are preferable and include the Makler chamber (Sefi Medical Instruments; 10 μm deep) and the Microcell chamber (Fertility Technologies, Inc.; 20 μm deep). Highly viscous specimens are best studied using the Makler chamber. If human spermatozoa are to be analysed during capacitation, and especially during motility hyperactivation, then a depth of 20 μm is acceptable for spermatozoa immediately after separation from the seminal plasma and resuspension in capacitation medium. For analyzing hyperactivation, the minimum acceptable depth should be greater. A depth of 50 μm is appropriate in this case and can be achieved using a Microcell chamber of this size. Alternatively, a depth of 50 μm can be achieved using a flat capillary tube of this vertical dimension (Vitro Dynamics, Inc.).

In current computer-aided sperm analysis of human semen, the spermatozoa are observed using positive phase-contrast optics, generally at a magnification of $67 \times$ ($10 \times$ objective lens and $6.7 \times$ ocular lens). The manufacturer will recommend the specific microscope requirements. When the spermatozoa are observed after separation from the seminal plasma, negative phase-contrast optics of the same magnification provides sperm images of improved clarity. This requires the use of a negative phase-contrast objective lens, but all other optical components are the same as for traditional positive phase-contrast optics.

XX.2 **Video recording of the semen for computer-aided sperm analysis**
It is recommended that a video tape recording be made of the living spermatozoa and that computer-aided sperm analysis be performed of this recording rather than directly from the video camera. This improves standardization and allows implementation of quality assurance procedures (see Chapter 5). The user should refer to the manufacturer regarding the choice of video tape recorder. Incorporation of a video time generator or similar coding device is helpful, so that each specimen can receive a distinct numerical or alphanumeric code.

The light intensity on the microscope should be standardized while video recording, by means of the control knob or lever for the microscope light source. Illumination is improved if the voltage to the microscope is stable.

It is important that a set of microscope fields be recorded spanning the entire slide preparation while avoiding the edges of the preparation. At least 10 such fields should be videotaped, for 7–10 seconds each. In specimens with low sperm concentration, e.g., less than 10×10^6 spermatozoa/ml, as many as 20 fields may be necessary to achieve sampling of at least 100 motile sperm for analysis (see below). During videotaping, the sperm heads should be brought into focus, and the illumination adjusted on the microscope to achieve maximum contrast between the sperm heads and the background.

XX.3 Use of the CASA instrument

The manufacturer's instructions should be carefully followed when setting up the CASA instrument. It should be maintained in a clean, dust-free environment in which there is minimum temperature fluctuation. Particular attention should be paid to the 'thresholding' step, which adjusts the luminosity of the CASA image prior to analysis. Other important steps include calibration of the image magnification, specification of the allowable size of the image of the sperm head, and adjustment of parameters to allow for the range of velocities of motile sperm. Here it is important to distinguish between the settings used in computing the percentage of motile sperm and those used in measuring individual sperm motion parameters. When the CASA instrument is prepared for each analysis session, the use of videotapes of semen specimens of several concentrations can provide a basis for quality control (Destefano *et al.*, 1989). These tapes could be made by each user or shared among users.

It is recommended that the CASA instrument be used to compute the movements of all sperm for an elapsed time of approximately half a second, at a video framing rate of 25–30 frames/second (depending upon the electrical standard of the country, and the subsequent adaptation of the CASA instrument). Sampling of all sperm for this time interval improves the accuracy and precision with which individual motion parameters are computed (Mack *et al.*, 1988). Shorter time intervals can reduce the accuracy with which measures of the pattern of sperm head motion are computed.

XX.4 CASA terminology

There is a standard terminology for parameters measured by CASA systems, some of which are illustrated in Fig. XX.1.

VCL = *curvilinear velocity* (μm/s). Time-average velocity of a sperm head along its actual curvilinear trajectory, as perceived in two dimensions under the microscope.

VSL = *straight-line velocity* (μm/s). Time-average velocity of a sperm head along the straight line between its first detected position and its last position.

VAP = *average path velocity* (μm/s). Time-average velocity of a sperm head along its spatial average trajectory. This trajectory is computed by smoothing the actual trajectory according to algorithms in the CASA instrument; these algorithms vary among instruments.

Fig. XX.1. Standard terminology for parameters measured by CASA systems.

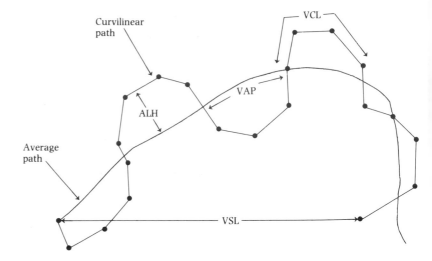

ALH = *amplitude of lateral head displacement* (μm). Magnitude of lateral displacement of a sperm head about its spatial average trajectory. It can be expressed as a maximum or an average of such displacements. Different CASA instruments compute ALH using different algorithms, so that values are not strictly comparable.

LIN = *linearity.* The linearity of a curvilinear trajectory, VSL/VCL.

WOB = *wobble.* Measure of oscillation of actual trajectory about its spatial average path, VAP/VCL.

STR = *straightness.* Linearity of the spatial average path, VSL/VAP.

BCF = beat/cross frequency (beats/s). The time-average rate at which the curvilinear sperm trajectory crosses its average path trajectory.

MAD = *mean angular displacement* (degrees). The time average of absolute values of the instantaneous turning angle of the sperm head along its curvilinear trajectory.

Different CASA instruments use different mathematical algorithms to compute many of these movement parameters. The degree of comparability of measurements across all instruments is not yet known. However, initial comparisons give relatively good agreement between some instruments (Davis & Katz, 1992).

XX.5 Statistical analysis

It is recommended that CASA analysis obtain movement parameters for at least 100 motile sperm tracks per specimen. Note that this will require detection of many more spermatozoa. If it is desired to sort sperm into subcategories of motion or to make other analyses of variability within a specimen, at least 200 motile tracks are necessary. Experimental designs should seek to standardize the number of sperm analysed per specimen. It is desirable to interface the CASA instruments with computer software that permits data organization and statistical analysis. The specimen distributions of many of the movement parameters are not normal. Therefore it is recommended that the median, rather than the mean value, be used to summarize the central tendency of each movement parameter. Depending on the statistical analyses to be performed, it may be necessary to perform mathematical transformations of the parameters for single sperm prior to such analyses. In some instances, nonparametric statistical tests may be necessary.

References

Destefano, F., Annest, J.L., Kresnow, M., Schrader, S.M. & Katz, D.F. (1989) Semen characteristics of Vietnamese veterans. *Reproductive Toxicology*, 3:165—73.

Mack, S.O., Wolf, D.P. & Tash, J.S. (1988) Quantitation of specific parameters of motility in large numbers of human sperm by digital image processing. *Biology of Reproduction*. 38:270–81.

Vantman, D., Koukoulis, G., Dennison, L., Zinaman, M. & Sherins, R.J. (1988) Computer-assisted semen analysis: evaluation of method and assessment of the influence of sperm concentration on linear velocity determination. *Fertility and Sterility*. 49:510–16.

Appendix XXI

Suggested instructions to patients in preparation for the postcoital test

The postcoital test is performed as closely as possible to the time of ovulation when the cervical mucus is most receptive to sperm migration. This is one of the tests in the diagnosis of infertility.

The following instructions should be followed, as closely as possible in preparation for the postcoital test.

(i) You and your partner should abstain from intercourse for at least two days before the test.

(ii) Attend to your toilet needs before intercourse. It will be necessary not to do so for a few hours afterwards.

(iii) The most suitable day for your test is _ (day) _ (month) _____ (year). Intercourse should take place on this day according to your normal practice. (Keep a sanitary napkin within reach.)

(iv) After coitus, rest on your back for about 30 minutes with your knees bent to raise the hips and to prevent the loss of semen.

(v) Put on the sanitary napkin/pad in the usual manner to avoid leakage of semen.

(vi) Report to the clinic for the test at _____ (time), on _____ (day) _____ (month) _____ (year).

(vii) Do not remove the sanitary napkin/pad until the time of examination by the doctor.

SAMPLE RECORD FORM FOR CERVICAL MUCUS SCORING AND POSTCOITAL TEST

Date of last menstrual period

	Day	Month	Year

Daily cervical mucus score

	Day / Month	Day / Month	Day / Month	Day / Month
Date				
Day of cycle				
Volume				
Consistency				
Ferning				
Spinnbarkeit				
Cellularity				
Total score				
pH	.	.	.	.

Postcoital test

	Day	Month
Date		

Time after coitus (h)

	Vaginal pool	Exocervical pool	Endocervical pool
Sperm/mm³			

Motility (100 spermatozoa)

	Vaginal pool	Exocervical pool	Endocervical pool
(a) Rapid progression			
(b) Slow progression			
(c) Nonprogressive			
(d) Immotile			

93

Appendix XXII

Sperm–cervical mucus interaction: the capillary tube test

XXII.1   **Equipment**
Use of the capillary tube test in the clinical evaluation of cervical mucus penetration received great impetus from the work of Kremer (1965, 1980), and the principles of his methods remain valid today. The test measures the ability of spermatozoa to penetrate a column of cervical mucus in a capillary tube. Various types of capillary tubes have been used, but those with a rectangular cross-section are recommended. The specific procedure recommended here was introduced by Pandya et al. (1986) and is a simplified version of the procedure of Kroeks & Kramer (1980). The test uses a flat capillary tube, 10 cm long, and 3 mm by 0.3 mm in cross section. Such tubes can be obtained from Vitro Dynamics, Rockaway, NJ, USA. The tube should be marked at 1-cm intervals, using a fine-pointed indelible marking pen.

XXII.2   **Method**
Fresh semen, not older than one hour after ejaculation, should be used. Cervical mucus is aspirated into a capillary tube, making sure that no air bubbles are introduced. The filling of the tube can be accomplished using a simple loading manifold made by filling the large end of a Pasteur pipette with an elastic sealant such as silicone glue (Katz et al., 1980). A flat hole is made in the sealant, through which the flat capillary tube is then pushed. Suction is applied at the opposite end of the pipette while the open end of the flat tube is placed in a pool of mucus. The tube should be filled with enough mucus that the mucus meniscus is no more than 2–3 cm from the top of the tube. Trailing mucus is cut from the lower end of the tube, and the upper end of the tube is sealed with plasticine, modelling clay, or similar agents. Enough sealer should be applied that the mucus column projects slightly out of the open end of the tube. After loading, the tube should be checked under the

microscope for the presence of spermatozoa in the mucus. If sperm are present, their numbers and motion should be assessed, so that a correction can be made in analysing the penetration of fresh sperm.

A small aliquot of well-mixed semen (50 μl) is pipetted into a reservoir container, such as a No. 00 BEEM capsule, and a slit is made in its cap to receive and support the capillary tube. Thus, the tube is in a vertical orientation during the period of sperm penetration. If the reservoir does not have a cap, then the tube should be supported to remain nearly vertical, and moist sponges or wipes should cover the opening of the reservoir. The temperature at which the test is performed should be standardized at 37 °C, and the reference results presented here are for that temperature.

XXII.3 Assessment of the test

This test focuses both on the migration distance of the penetrating sperm and on their density along the tube. This information is combined into a single quantitative score. After one hour of application of sperm to the mucus, the capillary tube is removed from the reservoir and the open end is rinsed with saline or, preferably, a mucolytic solution such as dithiotreitol (DTT, Sigma Catalogue No. D0632; 10 g/l) or mercaptoethanol, to remove residual spermatozoa from the mucus interface and surface of the tube. The tube is placed under a microscope and viewed using a $40 \times$ phase-contrast objective lens and $10 \times$ ocular lens. The numbers of spermatozoa are counted in three microscopic fields at the 1 cm, 4 cm and 7 cm marks along the tube. The total number of sperm in each group of three fields is determined, correcting for any initial sperm in the tube. This is expressed as the number per mm²), using the known microscope field area. This area can be calibrated using a stage micrometer. The position of the forward-most group of 'vanguard' spermatozoa is also noted. The results of the test are expressed as a rank score that has a maximum of 20. This is derived as the sum of the score for the numbers of spermatozoa/mm² at 1 cm, 4 cm, and 7 cm along the tube, plus the score for the position of the vanguard sperm. The following table summarizes the computation.

No. sperm/mm²	Score	Vanguard sperm	Score
0	0	less than 3 cm	0
1–30	1	≥ 3–< 4 cm	1
31–60	2	≥ 4–< 5 cm	2
61–120	3	≥ 5–< 6 cm	3
121–200	4	≥ 6–< 7 cm	4
> 200	5	≥ 7 cm	5

The result of the computation is then expressed according to the following table.

Total score	Result	Rank
0	Negative	0
1–8	Poor	1
9–11	Average	2
12–15	Good	3
16 or more	Excellent	4

References

Katz, D.F., Overstreet, J.W. & Hanson, F.W. (1980) A new quantitative test for sperm penetration into cervical mucus. *Fertility and Sterility.* **33**:179–86.

Kremer, J. (1965) A simple penetration test. *International Journal of Andrology.* **10**:209–15.

Kremer, J. (1980) *In vitro* sperm penetration in cervical mucus and AIH. In: *Homologous Artificial Insemination (AIH)*, ed. Emperaire, J.C., Audebert, A. & Hafez, E.S.E. The Hague, Martinus Nijhoff, pp. 30–7.

Kroeks, N.I. & Kremer, J (1980) The role of cervical factors in infertility. In *The Infertile Couple*, ed. Pepperell, R.J., Hudson, B. & Wood C. Edinburgh, Churchill-Livingstone, p. 112.

Pandya, I.J., Mortimer, D. & Sawers, R.S. (1986) A standardized approach for evaluating the penetration of human spermatozoa into cervical mucus in vitro. *Fertility and Sterility.* **45**:357–60.

Appendix XXIII

Standard procedure for counting cells and sperm in cervical mucus

Microscope slide preparations must be standardized to a known depth in order to perform objective counts of sperm or cell density. This can be achieved by supporting the coverglass with silicone grease (or other nonspermatotoxic material) impregnated with microspheres of the desired depth (Drobnis *et al.*, 1988). 'Posts' of grease can be placed at four positions on the slide, corresponding to the four corners of a coverglass (typically 22 mm × 22 mm). The sperm suspension, mucus, etc. is placed in the space within these posts, and the coverglass is then placed firmly upon them. The preparation can be sealed by pipetting mineral oil into the spaces between the posts. It is recommended that preparations containing cervical mucus be supported by grease with glass beads 100 μm in diameter (obtainable from Sigma Chemical Co; Catalogue No. G4649). These must be washed before mixing into the grease. The procedures are as follows.

Washing
Cover 150 ml of beads with acetone, swirl vigorously, and decant. Repeat two times.
Rinse 4–6 times with deionized water.
Cover with 1 M (mol/l) HCl, stir 20 minutes, then decant the acid.
Rinse 4–6 times with deionized water.
Cover with 2 M NaCl, stir 10 minutes, then decant the saline.
Rinse 2 times with 2 M NaCl.
Rinse 10 times with deionized water, stirring 2–5 minutes on each rinse.
Spread out beads in a Pyrex baking dish or other flat container and dry in an oven.
Beads may be autoclaved and stored under a sterile hood.

Preparation of supporting grease material

Empty approximately 10 ml of silicone grease (high vacuum grease, Dow Corning Corporation), or equivalent material, into a beaker.

Add approximately 2 ml of washed glass beads and mix thoroughly.

Remove the plunger from a 5- or 10-ml syringe (e.g., Sigma Chemical Co.). Using a weighing spatula, put as much of the grease material into the syringe as possible.

Replace the plunger, and with the nose of the syringe directed upward, push out as much air as possible.

Fit the syringe with a blunt, 10-gauge needle.

Counting sperm or other cells in the preparation

It is recommended that all sperm and cell counts be expressed in cells/mm^3. Calibration of the optical arrangement on any microscope can be performed using the following concepts. Traditional estimates of sperm or other cell density in cervical mucus have referred to the number of cells 'per high powered field' (HPF). The most common combination of microscopic optics to achieve this has been based upon a $40 \times$ objective lens and $10 \times$ standard field ocular lens (aperture size 14 mm), yielding a nominal magnification of $400 \times$. However, the size of the field viewed by an observer depends on the aperture size of the ocular lens. Modern microscopes are generally equipped with wide field oculars, thereby increasing the size of the field viewed. The diameter of the field observed is equal to the diameter of the aperture of the ocular lens divided by the magnification of the objective lens. A typical $10 \times$ wide-field ocular lens has an aperture of 20 mm. Thus, the diameter of the microscope field viewed with a $10 \times$ wide-field ocular and $40 \times$ objective lens is approximately 500 μm. If this field is 100 μm deep, its volume is then 0.02 mm^3. Thus, a count of 10 cells/HPF is equivalent to approximately 500 cells/mm^3 under these conditions.

References

Drobnis, E.Z., Yudin, A.L., Cherr, G.N. & Katz, D.F. (1988) Hamster sperm penetration of the zona pellucida: kinematic analysis and mechanical implications. *Developmental Biology*. **130**:311–23.

Appendix XXIV

Sperm preparation techniques

Procedures

Two simple preparation procedures are described based on the 'swim-up' of motile spermatozoa from semen and on discontinuous Percoll gradient centrifugation. For both techniques the culture medium suggested is supplemented Earle's, although other media such as Hams F10 are also appropriate.

XXIV.1 Swim-up

Supplemented Earle's medium (1.2 ml) is gently layered over semen (1 ml) in a sterile 15-ml conical-based centrifuge tube. The tube is inclined at an angle of 45° and incubated for 1 hour at 37 °C. It is then gently returned to the upright position and the uppermost 1 ml removed. This aliquot of motile cells is then diluted with 8 volumes of supplemented Earle's, centrifuged at 500g for 5 minutes, and finally resuspended in 0.5 ml of Earle's medium for the assessment of sperm concentration or sperm function, or for other procedures.

Constituents of supplemented Earle's medium
46 ml of Earle's balanced salt solution
4 ml of heat-inactivated (56 °C for 20 minutes) patient's serum
1.5 mg sodium pyruvate
0.18 ml sodium lactate
100 mg sodium bicarbonate

or

50 ml of Earle's balanced salt solution
300 mg bovine or human serum albumin[a]
1.5 mg sodium pyruvate
0.18 ml sodium lactate
100 mg sodium bicarbonate

[a]For assisted reproduction procedures such as *in vitro* fertilization (IVF), artificial insemination (AI), or gamete intrafallopian transfer (GIFT), it is imperative that the human serum albumin be highly purified and free from viral and bacterial contamination. Some preparations of albumin have been designed for such procedures (e.g., from Irvine Scientific, Santa Ana, CA, USA; Armour Pharmaceuticals, Eastbourne, United Kingdom).

XXIV.2 Discontinuous Percoll gradients

(i) 3 ml of 80% Percoll are pipetted into a 15-ml sterile, conical-bottomed tube.

(ii) 3 ml of 40% Percoll are gently pipetted on top of the 80% Percoll layer, care being taken not to disturb the interface between the two layers.

(111) 1–2 ml semen is then gently layered over the Percoll gradient and centrifuged at 500g for 20 minutes.

(iv) The pellet at the base of the 80% Percoll fraction is then resuspended in 5–10 ml of Earle's medium and centrifuged for 5 minutes at 500g before being resuspended in 1 ml of Earle's medium for the estimation of sperm concentration or sperm function, or for other procedures.

Constituents of isotonic Percoll
10 ml of 10× concentrated Earle's medium (e.g., from Flow Laboratories)
90 ml Percoll
300 mg bovine or human serum albumin[a] *or* 10 ml heat-inactivated patient's serum.
3 mg sodium pyruvate
0.37 ml sodium lactate (60% syrup)
200 mg sodium bicarbonate
Constituents of 80% Percoll
40 ml of isotonic Percoll
10 ml of supplemented Earle's medium
Constituents of 40% Percoll
20 ml of isotonic Percoll
30 ml of supplemented Earle's medium

XXIV.3 Preparation of poor quality samples

In cases of severe oligozoospermia and/or asthenozoospermia, Percoll gradients are preferable to the 'swim-up' method because of the improved recoveries obtained. Moreover the scale and composition of the Percoll gradient can be altered to meet the specific needs of individual samples. One possibility, for example, is to apply the sample to several mini-Percoll gradients (Ord *et al.*, 1990), containing only 0.3 ml volumes of the 40% and 80% Percoll fractions.

Reference

Ord, T. Patrizio, P., Marello, E., Balmaceda, J.P. & Asch, R.H. (1990) Mini-Percoll: a new method of semen preparation for IVF in severe male factor infertility. *Human Reproduction.* 5:987–9.

Appendix XXV

Basic requirements for an andrology laboratory

The following is a list of supplies and equipment that would enable a laboratory to perform the basic tests suggested in this manual and to function as an andrology laboratory. This assumes that a refrigerator, a centrifuge (swing-out rotor), and an incubator are already available.

A.   Safety of the andrology laboratory
1.   Rubber gloves
2.   Face masks
3.   Laboratory coats
4.   5.25 g/l sodium hypochlorite (e.g., household bleach diluted with 9 × its volume of water)
5.   Protective safety glasses
6.   First-aid kit
7.   Eye washing solution
8.   Shower (optional)

B.   Semen analysis
1.   WHO laboratory manual for the examination of human semen and sperm–cervical mucus interaction (third edition)
2.   Record forms for semen analysis
3.   Wide-mouth containers with lids (demonstrated not to have damaging effects on spermatozoa)
4.   Pasteur pipettes with latex droppers or plastic disposable transfer pipettes
5.   Automatic pipettes (e.g., Eppendorf, Oxford, Finnpipet, Pipetman, available from many suppliers)
6.   Positive displacement pipette to measure 50 μl, such as the Wiretrol II W-100 (Drummond Scientific Co., 500 Parkway,

Broomhall, PA 19008, USA); Chempette Series 7947-20 or 7947-30 (Cole-Parmer Instrument Co., 7425 North Oak Park Ave, Chicago, IL 60648-9830, USA); SMI Digital Adjust Micro/ Pettor Model P5068-20D (20 to 100μl) (SMI Liquid Handling Products, American Hospital Supply Corporation, Miami, FL 33152, USA)

7. Laboratory counter, such as the Clay Adams Lab Counter (Fisher Scientific, Springfield, NJ, USA, catalogue No. 02-670-13)
8. Haemocytometer (improved Neubauer)
9. Warming plate (bench top)
10. Vortex mixer
11. Phase-contrast microscope, to include $\times 10$, $\times 20$, $\times 40$ phase objectives, $\times 100$ oil-immersion objective, and $\times 10$ (wide-field) eyepiece
12. 50-watt light source

C. Sperm–cervical mucus interaction
1. Record forms for scoring
2. Mucus sampling syringe, e.g., Aspiglaire (BICEF, L'Aigle, France)
3. Rectangular glass capillary tubes for the capillary tube test, 3 mm width, 0.3 mm depth, 10 cm length (Microslide, Vitro Dynamics, Rockaway, NJ, USA)

D. Reagents for Immunobead or MAR test
See Appendices XI and XII

E. Clinical examination of a male patient with infertility
Orchidometer ('Test size' Remcat Trade AB, PO Box 5011, S-16205, Vallingby, Sweden)

Bibliography

Asterisk indicates review article

Aitken, R.J. & Clarkson, J.S. (1987) Cellular basis of defective sperm function and its association with genesis of reactive oxygen species by human spermatozoa. *Journal of Reproduction and Fertility.* **81**: 459-69.

Aitken, R.J. & Clarkson, J.S. (1988) Significance of reactive oxygen species in defining the efficacy of sperm preparation techniques. *Journal of Andrology.* **9**: 367–76.

Aitken, R.J., Clarkson, J.S. & Fishel, S. (1989) Generation of reactive oxygen species, lipid peroxidation and human sperm function. *Biology of Reproduction.* **41**: 183–7

Aitken, R.J., Irvine, D.S. & Wu, F.C.W. (1991) Prospective analysis of sperm-oocyte fusion and reactive oxygen species generation as criteria for the diagnosis of infertility. *American Journal of Gynecology.* **164**: 542–51.

Aitken, R.J., Thatcher, S., Glasier, A.F., Clarkson, J.S., Wu, F.C.W. & Baird, D.T. (1987) Relative ability of modified versions of the hamster oocyte penetration test, incorporating hyperosmotic medium or the ionophore A23187, to predict IVF outcome. *Human Reproduction.* **2**: 227–31.

Aitken, R.J. & West, K.M. (1990) Analysis of the relationship between reactive oxygen species production and leucocyte infiltration in fractions of human semen separated on Percoll gradients. *International Journal of Andrology.* **13**: 433–51.

Alvarez, J.G., Touchstone, J.C., Blasco, L. & Storey, B.T. (1987) Spontaneous lipid peroxidation and production of hydrogen peroxide and superoxide in human spermatozoa. Superoxide dismutase as major enzyme protectant against oxygen toxicity. *Journal of Andrology.* **8**: 338–48.

Ayvaliotis, B., Bronson, R., Rosenfeld, D. & Cooper, G. (1985) Conception rates in couples where autoimmunity to sperm is detected. *Fertility and Sterility.* **43**: 739–42.

Barratt, C.L.R., Bolton, A.E. & Cooke, I.D. (1990) Functional significance of white blood cells in the male and female reproductive tract. *Human Reproduction.* **5**: 639–44.

Berger, T., Marrs, R.P. & Moyer, D.L. (1985) Comparison of techniques for selection of motile spermatozoa. *Fertility and Sterility.* **43**: 268–73.

Bland, J.M. & Altman, D.G. (1986) Statistical methods for assessing agreement between two methods of clinical measurement. *Lancet.* **I**: 307–10

*Boyers, S.P., Davis, R.O. & Katz, D.F. (1989) Automated semen analysis. *Current Problems in Obstetrics, Gynaecology and Fertility.* Chicago, IL, Year Book Medical Publishers, Inc. **XII**: 173–200.

103

*Bronson, R.A., Cooper, G.W. & Rosenfeld, D. (1984) Sperm antibodies: their role in infertility. *Fertility and Sterility.* **42**: 171–83.

Brunner, H., Weidner, W. & Schiefer, H.G. (1983) Studies on the role of *Ureaplasma urealyticum* and *Mycoplasma hominis* in prostatitis. *Journal of Infectious Diseases.* **147**: 807–13.

Burkman, L.J., Kruger, T.F., Coddington, C.C., Rosenwaks, Z., Franken, D.R. & Hodgen, G.D. (1988) The hemizona assay (HZA): development of a diagnostic test for the binding of human spermatozoa to human hemizona pellucida to predict fertilization potential. *Fertility and Sterility.* **49**: 688–97.

Clarke, G.N., Elliott, P.J. & Smaila, C. (1985) Detection of sperm antibodies in semen using the Immunobead test: a survey of 813 consecutive patients. *American Journal of Reproductive Immunology and Microbiology.* **7**: 118–23.

Comhaire, F., Verschraegen, G. & Vermeulen, L. (1980) Diagnosis of accessory gland infection and its possible role in male infertility. *International Journal of Andrology.* **3**: 32–45.

Cross, N.L., Morales, P., Overstreet, J.W. & Hanson, F.W. (1986). Two simple methods for detecting acrosome-reacted human sperm. *Gamete Research.* **15**: 213–26.

Cummins, J.M., Pember, S.M., Jequier, A.M., Yovich, J.L. & Hartmann, P.E. (1991) A test of the human sperm acrosome reaction following ionophore challenge: Relationship to fertility and other seminal parameters. *Journal of Andrology.* **12**: 98–103.

*Davis, R.O. & Katz, D.F. (1992) Standardization and comparability of CASA instruments. *Journal of Andrology.* **13**: 81–6.

Davis, R.O. Rothmann, S.A. & Overstreet, J.W. (1992). Accuracy and precision of computer-aided sperm analysis in multicenter studies. *Fertility and Sterility.* **57**: 648–53.

Drevius, L. & Eriksson, H. (1966) Osmotic swelling of mammalian spermatozoa. *Experimental Cell Research.* **42**: 136–56.

Dunphy, B.C., Kay R., Barratt, C.L.R. & Cooke, I.D. (1989) Quality control during the conventional analysis of semen, an essential exercise. *Journal of Andrology.* **10**: 378–85.

Egozcue, J., Templado, C., Vidal, F., Navarro, J., Morer-Fargas, F. & Marina, S. (1983) Meiotic studies in a series of 1100 infertile and sterile males. *Human Genetics.* **65**: 185–8.

Gagnon, C. (ed.) (1990). *Controls of Sperm Motility: Biological and Clinical Aspects.* Boca Raton, CRC Press.

Gellert-Mortimer, S.T., Clarke, G.N., Baker, H.W.G., Hyne, R.V. & Johnson, W.I.H. (1988) Evaluation of Nycodenz and Percoll density gradients for the selection of motile human spermatozoa. *Fertility and Sterility.* **49**: 335–41.

Ginsberg, K.A. & Armant, D.R. (1990) The influence of chamber characteristics on the reliability of sperm concentration and movement measurements obtained by manual and videomicrographic analysis. *Fertility and Sterility.* **53**: 882–7.

Harris, S.J., Milligan, M.P., Masson, G.M. & Dennis, K.J. (1981) Improved separation of motile sperm in asthenozoospermia and its application to artificial insemination homologous (AIH). *Fertility and Sterility.* **36**: 219–21.

Hellstrom, W.J.G., Samuels, S.J., Waits, A.B. & Overstreet J.W. (1989) A comparison of the usefulness of SpermMar and Immunobead tests for the detection of antisperm antibodies. *Fertility and Sterility.* **52**: 1027–31.

Hill, J.A., Haimovici, F., Politch, J.A. & Anderson, D.J. (1987) Effects of soluble products of activated lymphocytes and macrophages (lymphokines and monokines) on human sperm motion parameters. *Fertility and Sterility.* **47**: 460–5.

Huszar, G., Corrales, M. & Vigue, L. (1988) Correlation between sperm creatine phosphokinase activity and sperm concentrations in normospermic and oligozoospermic men. *Gamete Research.* **19**: 67–75.

Huszar, G., Vigue, L. & Corrales, M. (1990) Sperm creatine kinase activity in fertile and infertile oligozoospermic men. *Journal of Andrology.* **11**: 40–6.

Insler, V., Melmed, H., Eichenbrenner, I., Serr, D.M. & Lunnenfeld, B. (1972) The cervical score. A simple semiquantitative method for monitoring of the menstrual cycle. *International Journal of Gynaecology and Obstetrics.* **10**: 223–28.

Jeyendran, R.S., Van der Ven, H.H., Perez-Pelaez, M. Crabo, B.G. & Zaneveld, L.J.D. (1984) Development of an assay to assess the functional integrity of the human sperm membrane and its relationship to the other semen characteristics. *Journal of Reproduction and Fertility.* **70**: 219–28.

*Jones, W.R. (1986) Immunological factors in infertility. In *The Infertile Couple*, ed. Pepperell, R.J., Hudson, B. and Wood, C. Edinburgh, Churchill Livingstone (2nd edition).

Jones, R., Mann, T. & Sherins, R. (1979) Peroxidative breakdown of phospholipids by human spermatozoa, spermicidal properties of fatty acid perodixes and protective action of seminal plasma. *Fertility and Sterility.* **31**: 531–7.

Jouannet, P., Ducot, B., Feneux, D. & Spira, A. (1988) Male factors and the likelihood of pregnancy in infertile couples. I. Study of sperm characteristics. *International Journal of Andrology.* **11**: 379–94.

Katz, D.F., Overstreet, J.W., Samuels, S.J., Niswander, P.W., Bloom, T.D. & Lewis, E.L. (1986) Morphometric analysis of spermatozoa in the assessment of human male fertility. *Journal of Andrology.* **7**: 203–10.

Katz, D.F., Drobnis, E.Z. & Overstreet, J.W. (1989) Factors regulating mammalian sperm migration through the female reproductive tract and oocyte investments. *Gamete Research.* **22**: 443–69.

Katz, D.F., Morales, P., Samuels, S.J. & Overstreet, J.W. (1990) Mechanisms of filtration of morphologically abnormal human sperm by cervical mucus. *Fertility and Sterility.* **54**: 513–6.

Knuth, U.A., Neuwinger, J. & Nieschlag, E. (1989) Bias of routine semen analysis by uncontrolled changes in laboratory environment: detection by long term sampling of monthly means for quality control. *International Journal of Andrology.* **12**: 375–83.

Kremer, J. & Jager, S. (1980) Characteristics of anti-spermatozoal antibodies responsible for the shaking phenomenon, with special regard to immunoglobulin class and antigen-reactive sites. *International Journal of Andrology.* **3**: 143–52.

*Krieger, J.N. (1984) Prostatitis syndrome: pathophysiology, differential diagnosis and treatment. *Sexually Transmitted Diseases.* **11**: 100–12.

Lessley, B.A. & Garner, D.L. (1983) Isolation of motile spermatozoa by density gradient centrifugation in Percoll. *Gamete Research.* **7**: 49–61.

Liu, D.Y., Lopata, A., Johnston, W.H.I. & Baker, H.W.G. (1988) A human sperm-zona pellucida binding test using oocytes that failed to fertilize in-vitro. *Fertility and Sterility.* **50**: 782–8.

Liu, D.Y., Clarke, G.Y., Lopata, A., Johnson, W.I.H. & Baker, H.W.G. (1989) A sperm-zona pellucida binding test and in-vitro fertilization. *Fertility and Sterility.* **50**: 281–7.

Lopata, A., Patullo, M.J., Chang, A. & James, B. (1976) A method for collecting motile spermatozoa from human semen. *Fertility and Sterility.* **27**: 677–84.

Lorton, S.P., Kummerfeld, H.L. & Foote, R.H. (1981) Polyacrylamide as a substitute for cervical mucus in sperm migration tests. *Fertility and Sterility.* **35**: 222–5.

Makler, A. (1980) The improved ten-micrometer chamber for rapid sperm count and motility evaluation. *Fertility and Sterility.* **33**: 337–8.

Makler, A., Murillo, O., Huszar, G., Tarlatzis, B., DeCherney, A. & Naftolin, F. (1984) Improved techniques for collecting motile spermatozoa from human semen. I. A self-migratory method. *International Journal of Andrology.* **7**: 61–70.

Meares, E.M. & Stamey, T.A. (1972) The diagnosis and management of bacterial prostatitis. *British Journal of Urology.* **44**: 175–9.

Mobley, D.F. (1975) Semen cultures in the diagnosis of bacterial prostatitis. *Journal of Urology.* **114**: 83–5.

Moghissi, K.S. (1976) Post-coital test: physiological basis, technique and interpretation. *Fertility and Sterility.* **27**: 117–29.

Moghissi, K.S. (1986) Evaluation and management of cervical hostility. *Seminars in Reproductive Endocrinology.* **4**: 343–55.

Mortimer, D., Leslie, E.E., Kelly, R.W. & Templeton, A.A. (1982) Morphological selection of human spermatozoa in vivo and in vitro. *Journal of Reproduction and Fertility.* **64**: 391–9.

Mortimer, D. (1985). The male factor in infertility. Part 1. Semen analysis. In: *Current Problems in Obstetrics, Gynaecology and Fertility,* ed. J.M. Leventhal, Chicago, IL, Year Book Medical Publishers, Inc., pp. 1–87.

Mortimer, D., Shu, M.A. & Tan, R. (1986) Standardization and quality control of sperm concentration and sperm motility counts in semen analysis. *Human Reproduction.* **1**: 299–303.

*Mortimer, D. (1990) Objective analysis of sperm motility and kinematics. In: *Handbook of the Laboratory Diagnosis and Treatment of Infertility,* ed. B.A. Keel & B.W. Webster, Boca Raton, CRC Press, pp. 97–133.

Mortimer, D., Curtis, E.F. & Camenzind, A.R. (1990a) Combined use of fluorescent peanut agglutinin lectin and Hoechst 33258 to monitor the acrosomal status and vitality of human spermatozoa. *Human Reproduction.* **5**: 99–103.

Mortimer, D., Mortimer, S.T., Shu, M.A. & Swart, R. (1990b) A simplified approach to sperm-cervical mucus interaction testing using a hyaluronate migration test. *Human Reproduction.* **5**: 835–41.

Neuwinger, J., Behre, H. & Nieschlag, E. (1990) External quality control in the andrology laboratory: an experimental multicenter trial. *Fertility and Sterility.* **54**: 308–14.

Oehninger, S., Burkman, L.J., Coddington, C.C., Acosta, A.A., Scott, R., Franken, D.A. & Hodgen, G.D. (1989) Hemizona assay: assessment of sperm dysfunction and prediction of in-vitro fertilization outcome. *Fertility and Sterility.* **51**: 665–70.

Pattinson, H.A. & Mortimer, D. (1987) Prevalence of sperm surface antibodies in the male partners of infertile couples as determined by Immunobead screening. *Fertility and Sterility.* **48**: 466–9.

Purvis, K., Rui, H., Scholberg, A., Hesla, S. & Clausen, O.P.F. (1990) Application of flow cytometry to studies on the human acrosome. *Journal of Andrology.* **11**: 361–6.

Rao, B., Soufir, J.C., Martin, M. & David, G. (1989) Lipid peroxidation in human spermatozoa as related to midpiece abnormalities and motility. *Gamete Research.* **24**: 127–34.

Scarselli, G., Livi, C., Chelo, E., Dubini, V. & Pellagrini S. (1987) Approach to immunological male infertility: a comparison between MAR test and direct immunobead test, *Acta Europea Fertilitatis.* **18**: 55–9.

Serafini, P., Blank, W., Tran, C., Mansourian, M., Tan, T, & Batzofin, J. (1990) Enhanced penetration of zona-free hamster ova by sperm prepared by Nycodenz and Percoll gradient centrifugation. *Fertility and Sterility.* **53**: 551–5.

Urry, R.L., Middleton, R.G., McNamara, L. & Vikari, C.A. (1983) The effect of single density bovine serum albumin columns on sperm concentration, motility and morphology. *Fertility and Sterility.* **40**: 666–9.

Weidner, W., Krause, W., Scheifer, H.G., Brunner, H. & Friedrich, H.J. (1985) Ureaplasmal infections of the male urogenital tract, in particular prostatitis and semen quality. *Urologia Internationalis.* **40**: 5–9.

Wikland, M., Wik, O., Steen, Y., Quist, K., Söderlund, B. & Jansen, P.O. (1987) A self-migration method for preparation of sperm for *in vitro* fertilization. *Human Reproduction.* **2**: 191–5.

Wolff, H. & Anderson, D.J. (1988*a*) Immunohistological characterization and quantitation of leukocyte subpopulations in human semen. *Fertility and Sterility.* **49**: 497–504.

Wolff, H. & Anderson, D.J. (1988*b*) Evaluation of granulocyte elastase as a seminal plasma marker for leukocytospermia. *Fertility and Sterility.* **50**: 129–32.

Wolff, H., Politch, J.A., Martinez, A., Haimovici, F., Hill, J.A. & Anderson, D.J. (1990) Leukocytospermia is associated with poor semen quality. *Fertility and Sterility.* **53**: 528–36.

World Health Organization. (1983) *Laboratory Biosafety Manual.* Geneva, pp. 1–123.

World Health Organization. (1986). Consultation on: The zona-free hamster oocyte penetration test and the diagnosis of male fertility. ed. R.J. Aitken. *International Journal of Andrology (Supplement 6).*

World Health Organization Task Force on Methods for the Regulation of Male Fertility. (1990) Contraceptive efficacy of testosterone-induced azoospermia in normal men. *Lancet.* **336**: 995–9.

Yanagimachi, R., Lopata, A., Odom, C.B., Bronson, R.A., Mahi, C.A. & Nicolson, A.L. (1979) Retention of biologic characteristics of zona pellucida in highly concentrated salt solution: the use of salt stored eggs for assessing the fertilizing capacity of spermatozoa. *Fertility and Sterility.* **31**: 562–74.

Zavos, P.M. (1985) Seminal parameters of ejaculates collected from oligospermic and normospermic patients via masturbation and at intercourse with the use of Silastic seminal fluid collection device. *Fertility and Sterility.* **44**: 517–20.

de Ziegler, D., Cedars, M.I., Hamilton, F., Moreno, T. & Meldrum, D.R. (1987) Factors influencing maintenance of sperm motility during in vitro processing. *Fertility and Sterility.* **48**: 816–20.